Dental Care in Society

The Sociology of Dental Health

by
Marcel A. Fredericks
Ralph R. Lobene
and
Paul Mundy

McFarland & Company, Inc., Publishers
Jefferson, North Carolina 1980

Library of Congress Cataloging in Publication Data

Fredericks, Marcel A 1927-
Dental care in society.

Bibliography: p.
Includes index.
1. Dentistry—Social aspects. 2. Dental Care—Social aspects. I. Lobene, Ralph R., 1924- joint author. II. Mundy, Paul, 1919- joint author. III. Title. [DNLM: 1. Dentistry. 2. Sociology. WU100 F852d]
RK52.5.F73 362.1'976 80-15985
ISBN 0-89950-001-3

to

Janet, Lucille, and Mary Kay

Whose sacrifices and help
have made this volume
a reality

Acknowledgments

Our thanks are extended to all the students whom we have taught both nationally and internationally at the undergraduate and graduate levels. To the students at Loyola University School of Medicine, Forsyth Dental Center, Harvard University Medical School, Loyola University School of Dentistry, and Loyola University School of Nursing, we are grateful for their thought-provoking comments and questions about dental care during our lectures on the health care institution.

The authors are most grateful to Catherine O'Connell for her painstaking efforts with the manuscript. Her editorial contributions to this volume are appreciated. We appreciate too the services of Mr. Adegbola Adejunmobi on this project as research assistant in the Loyola University Department of Sociology.

Also at Loyola, we wish to thank Fr. Raymond C. Baumhart, S.J., president, Dr. Richard A. Matré, vice-president, and Dr. Raffaele Suriano, dean of the School of Dentistry, for their valuable statements made concerning health care and dental education over the past decade. Some of their comments are incorporated in this volume.

We happily acknowledge our debt to Dr. Ronald E. Walker, dean of the College of Arts and Sciences; Fr. Thomas M. Gannon, S.J., chairman of the Department of Sociology; Mrs. Helen Bruce, director of the Grant Information Office; and Mrs. Lucille McGill, administrative assistant in the Department of Sociology.

Our gratitude is extended to Dr. Louis Blanchet and Dr. Raymond Warpeha, who offered valuable insights over the years on the interrelationships of sociological variables and dental health care.

We also wish to acknowledge and give credit to John B. Sanders for the photographs appearing in this volume.

To Janet Paulsen, Sylvia Rdzak, Anna McLean and Reid S. Jacobson, we are grateful for their assistance in rereading the final draft of the manuscript.

In a special way, Dr. Fredericks wishes to extend his thanks to Dr. Joel J. Alpert, the late Dr. John Kosa, and his many colleagues during his U.S. Public Health Service post-doctoral fellowship years of research and teaching at the Harvard University Medical School.

Table of Contents

Foreword

Historically, the social sciences and dentistry have enjoyed a flirtatious relationship with each other, characterized by a superficial interaction without a longstanding and deep commitment. Each year the social scientists admit that it is getting better, and it is, but there is a continuing need to document the literature base and to provide educators and clinicians with comparative data on the interlocking systems of social, cultural, and psychological determinants relative to dentistry and dental health.

The present book is the first published attempt to inform the dental profession in a comprehensive and cohesive fashion about the societal components which influence health care delivery, preventive practices and disease rates. It discusses basic sociological concepts which all practitioners of the healing arts must contemplate to effectively render care, and to understand and modify patients' behavior.

The topics chosen by the authors reflect an interesting mix of theoretical concerns and actual studies of health care delivery systems, from the larger systems of government and bureaucracy to the small organizational structures of private practice and the interaction between members of the dental health team. They have explored the dimensions of the impact of the family on health and disease, a topic which has been neglected critically in the literature and in research studies in general. And yet, the American family (in all of its modern variable forms) is probably the most important change agent in the whole process of oral health.

The book stresses the need for an analysis of community

forces which should be considered in introducing changes in beliefs and behaviors. The influence of conflicts in cultural (ethnic) values and failure to implement health programs has been well-documented in the literature. This sociological study further focuses on social class, socioeconomic status, and race and their relationship to whether and to what degree people seek and/or find dental health care.

Dental care provided by a team in private practice and by the community at large is discussed from a sociological point of view by an examination of communication skills in small and large groups, in hospitals, for the aged (as a social phenomenon), and the social and scientific controversy surrounding fluoride. Urban and rural differences in health care delivery, and in attitudes toward health maintenance are skillfully here presented, bringing the sociological framework to bear on a clearer definition of the "geography of oral disease."

Dentistry is a people-intensive profession and health care delivery involves more than the reduction of disease through technological means or the better delivery of health care by effective organization. It involves a blending of those components with humanism; with a consideration of the values, norms and folkways of individuals and groups, and of concern about the inner person, his or her immediate and extended social network, and the larger culture.

This book will serve as the standard sociological text for dental and dental auxiliary educators and health professionals in general, offering as it does a firm basis for understanding the influence of social sciences on dentistry, and joining as it does the two bases of knowledge in a commitment to each other.

Patricia P. Cormier
Associate Dean for Academic Affairs
School of Dental Medicine
University of Pennsylvania

Chapter 1

Society-Culture-Personality and Dental Health Care

In the past, social scientists have contributed much to the fields of medicine, dentistry, and nursing. At present, the behavioral sciences have been accorded an important, even vital, place in the education of future physicians, dentists, nurses, dental auxiliaries and other health care professionals. With the inclusion of behavioral sciences components in the National Board Examination (1972), many medical schools have revised their curricula to include sociology in the training of future physicians. In dentistry, the behavioral sciences group of the International Association for Dental Research has increased in membership over the past years. However, the tremendous shortage of qualified social scientists has made it difficult to meet the needs of dental schools and dental auxiliary programs. In view of this problem, our attempt in this volume will be to present a synopsis of selected sociological concepts insofar as these bear on the education of future dental health care professionals. This volume is especially adapted to the needs of dental students, dental auxiliaries, dental practitioners, and dental administrators, who have not been fully introduced to the behavioral sciences.

Society, culture and *personality* form an interlocking social system. Change in any one of these components will, of necessity, affect the others—and thus the system.

Society may be defined as "an ordered and dynamic system of all the social interactions involving the members (personalities) of a total population, which can be identified as sharing a culture distinct from that shared by other populations."[1]*

**References will be found beginning on page 147.*

2 Dental Care

The two basic elements necessary for a society are a number of individuals and the existence of the group over a long period of time. Adaptation and organization of the behavior of the individual members of the group lead to development of a group consciousness, a feeling of unity, an esprit de corps. This process begins with a division of activities and their assignment to certain individuals, and is paralleled by the development of a community of ideas, values, and habits, or a psychological unit. When a group has reduced its members' cooperation to habitual voluntary patterns and has developed an esprit de corps, it is classified as a society.

All societies, however large or small, have a culture of their own—the society's way of life, or the things that the members of society think, feel, and do. Culture includes socially transmitted knowledge, beliefs, customs, laws, and habits—besides the artifacts of a people.

Culture has a three-fold function: It serves to adapt man to his physical environment through technology, to his social group through social organization, and to the supernatural world through religion and magic. General experiences are the same for one particular culture, but differ from culture to culture. As one grows older, experiences are more numerous and more complex. Thus every society exercises a series of influences upon its growing members. Although these influences have an effect on personality, they do not make the particular personality.

Society and culture, to some people, seem to be overlapping or identical; however, they are distinct though interrelated. Society is an organized group of people, a collection of individuals who have lived and worked together. Culture, on the other hand, is an organized group of psychic and material items, of behavior patterns. Society and culture persist through time and are largely self-perpetuating. The perpetuation of society and culture is based upon learning; the individuals born into the society are trained to occupy particular places in the social system. The success of the training depends upon a standardization of behavior of the society's members; these behavior standards are called cultural patterns.[2] A cultural pattern by definition is a consensus of behavior or opinion. It represents a mode of consistency in the behavior of members of that group in response to what they consider similar situations.

The term culture may also be used to refer to patterns of behavior which characterize human subgroups within specific societies. When the word is used in this way, it is often modified into *subculture*. There are "occupational subcultures, for example, which distinguish military, medical or railroad families from other people in the same society; ethnic or racial subcultures among native-born American blacks, Italians, or Mexican-Americans; illegal subcultures of crime and politics and so on."[3] Health care professionals share the general American culture into which they were born but they also share the behavioral traits only with each other which have been developed through the period of their training.[4]

As the culture of a society is incorporated by the individual person, a personality which is unique and distinctive to that person and also more or less adjusted to the demands of society is developed. Personality then is the dynamic system of ideas, attitudes, habits, and values (internalized from the *culture* and mediated through society) which are unique to the individual person.

The genetic (or *natural*) basis for personality is the combination of traits that results from the person's unique constellation of genes. However, this genetic basis represents only potentiality. These potentialities, when developed under the influence of the total environment in which an individual's orientation takes place, are shaped into a personality. Hence, the formation of the personality is one integrating the individual's experience with his physical qualities to form a mutually adjusted functioning whole. This takes place mainly in childhood and adolescence, and results in the development of distinctive physical as well as emotional responses.

The formal relations of the individual with other members of his society are controlled by his culture. Socialization is achieved through interaction. Socialization, or learning, occurs in a social environment, which is influenced by the values of the individual's culture.

It is important that the dental health care professional recognize the implications of the *society-culture-personality* system for the diagnosis, treatment and prognosis of a patient. To be understood properly, beliefs and attitudes toward health and illness must be examined in a societal and cultural context. Since these beliefs and attitudes are strongly ingrained in each individual, the health care practitioner must be able to utilize his or her knowledge of cultural variations in an individual's perceptions of health and illness, in order for patient care to be effective.[5]

Saunders[6] notes that in the Southwest, "Anglos" and Spanish-speaking persons had different attitudes toward illness. "Anglos" preferred modern science and hospitalization, while the Spanish-speaking Americans relied heavily on family care and support as well as folk medicine. In Guyana, many villagers of African and East Indian background would use the stem of the black sage tree in place of a tooth brush. They would break a limb off the black sage tree (which grows wild in the countryside) and make a brush of it by grinding one side with their teeth. The juices which result from the process seem to have a protective effect on the dentine and gums of the villagers. After the teeth and gums are cleaned, the black sage brush is bent in semi-circle fashion and the individual scrapes the tongue. After this is completed, the brush is disposed of; this cycle is repeated each morning before breakfast.

Culture and dental illnesses are clearly related. It has been asserted that "disease never comes haphazardly ... it always reflects the circumstances of our lives ... dental decays, cancer of the lungs, beri-beri, and innumerable other ailments are very precise indicators of the things we use, eat, do or lack."[7] Within this context, diet is a significant factor in the cause of dental caries. A poor diet may result in a decline in the health of the oral cavity and dental decay is a manifestation of such decline.[8]

In a different analysis of the way in which a group's cultural values are related to health, Zborowski[9] has attempted to specify the varying cultural orientations toward pain among persons in different ethnic groups. Zborowski notes that, in general, Italians consider pain as a physical misery to be complained about, to be relieved immediately and then forgotten. Jewish patients, on the contrary, often regard it as something to be complained about, but also to be worried about in relation to the significance for one's future and the future of one's family. "Old American" patients try to take a "detached and unemotional view of their symptoms." These individuals view pain as something not to be complained about, but to be relieved scientifically with an optimistic expectation regarding the outcome.

Public health workers must often make use of resourceful strategies when confronted with cultural beliefs harmful to health, and must invent artful detours. For example, Allport[10] cites the dilemma of one health educator in Zululand who found that milk was badly needed in the diets of expectant and nursing mothers. Because the belief system excluding the partaking of cow's milk was too deep to combat, the health educator prescribed the substitution of powdered milk in the diet, which met no resistance. The health of the women was therefore greatly improved.

In short, personal definitions of and responses to health, disease, and pain are molded by the sociocultural context of the patients in which they occur.

The influence of culture upon illness, health care and health can be appreciated only if the significance of culture is really understood. Once the impact of culture is grasped, its relationship to sickness and health is obvious. An example to show that public and professional attitudes toward health are a function of cultural values is seen in the relative emphasis in medical and dental specializations between pediatrics and pedodontics on the one hand and geriatrics (including dental care for the aged) on the other. To a large degree, the American culture values youth. Hence, the emphasis placed upon youth could be a contributing factor as to why the specialities of pediatrics and pedodontics are well established in contrast to the speciality of geriatrics which is underdeveloped.

It has been noted that society, culture and personality form an interlocking social system. By definition, a social system is a patterned relationship of statuses and roles. A society is the most inclusive form of a social system; it may contain many other subsystems (groups) as constituent parts. Status refers to a position in society; role is the dynamic aspect of status. Moreover, a role is the pattern of behavior expected of a person who occupies a particular status. There are two categories of status. These are ascribed status, which is derived from attributes over which the individual has no control such as age, sex, color, race, and nationality, and cannot be changed, and achieved status, that which an individual attains as the result of his or her own efforts in society.

In complex societies such as the United States, Britain, and France, a given individual has to play several roles, sometimes alternating from one to another quite rapidly. A woman may play the role of hygienist in her working hours; at home she plays the role of wife and mother, while in her leisure hours she divides her time between shopping and playing tennis with neighbors. At times, most people are not conscious that they are playing a role; as Goffman has pointed out, some are able to detach themselves from the role. Such detachment he calls "role distance." The social system, therefore, can be seen as a network of statuses, each with its appropriate role waiting to be played by individuals within the system.

Society-Culture-Personality and Institutions

As statuses and roles become highly complex structures, they are called institutions—*i.e.*, ways of taking care of (or striving to take care of) basic humans needs. Since people live together, they also develop social needs, which are often referred to as derived needs. Whereas the biological needs are the needs of the individual, derived needs are the needs of the group. If the institutions which provide for these needs were not available, then society would not be able to exist. For example, all societies must have institutions of socialization and education by which they transmit their culture to new members. Social institutions are crescive in nature and have a strain of consistency, which simply means that they develop over time and are interrelated. Institutions must exist for the maintenance of health and the treatment of illness. In simple societies these tend to be primarily magical and religious in orientation.

Health care is one of the vital institutions of American society and one of the most formal. The ceremonials which are part of the dentist's or physician's office attest to this process of formalization. Health care as an institution cannot be fully understood unless it is examined by itself as well as in relation to other institutions such as the family, religion, education, government, the economy, the recreation sphere, social welfare, science, and others.

For example, if we examine the institution of the family in relation to the health care institution we see that it is very important for a dental health care professional to be aware of the particular social class, age, racial, ethnic, family, and religious background of a patient. Gonda[11] notes that a significant relationship was observed between persistent complaints of pain and the patient's age and family background. Both older people and those from large families were more likely to be persistent complainers.

Indeed, it makes a difference whether the family is dependent or nondependent. Dependent families are less likely to visit a physician or a dentist regularly, and yet are more likely to utilize public medical and dental facilities.

The interrelationships of institutions can be seen if one examines education and health care. Depending upon social class, patients' educational backgrounds will differ; the level of education, in turn, affects the ease with which a patient and a health care professional can communicate. Skipper and Mumford[12] indicate that the "lower the educational attainment of the patient, the greater the possibility that this obstacle [fear of the physician or dentist] will be a problem and the problem is compounded by limited vocabulary.... Physicans [and dentists] may offer explanations to patients, but the message does not get through because the patient is unable to interpret the medical [or dental] vocabulary." Further Koos[13] asserts that upper-class persons are more likely than lower-class persons to view themselves as ill when they have particular symptoms. When questioned about specific symptoms, they reported more frequently than the lower classes that they would seek a doctor's advice.

Thus the institutions of education and the family bear important relationships and implications to the health care institution. Indeed, patients do not stand alone but are members of families and they react and behave in terms of the influence that their family—the most basic agency of the socialization process—has had on their understanding of and attitudes toward health and disease.

Therefore it is important to note that the tasks involved in these institutions of family and education are shared increasingly with other institutions—governmental, religious, recreational and economic. Thus societal needs are met by several institutions working together, and the more complex the society, the more dependent one institution is likely to be upon another.

Values, Norms, Folkways

Institutions can also be described as socially approved patterns of behavior. In examining this definition of institutions, the concepts of values, norms, folkways and mores become most important. A value is a social judgment, goal or activity that is important to an individual or group. Values are the "criteria or conceptions used in evaluating things (including objects, ideas, acts, feelings, and events) as to their relative desirability or merit. Values define what is good, beautiful, moral, and worthwhile."[14] Examples of values are justice, freedom, patriotism and love. When these generalized standards of behavior are expressed in more concrete forms, they are said to be norms, that is, rules for behavior. Norms include morality, custom, etiquette, usages and law. The term norm refers to a code of behavior to which people are expected to conform and does *not* refer to how people actually behave in society. From birth the individual begins to learn the norms of his society. He learns how he is expected to behave as a result of contact, first with his parents and other adults and later with other children.

To explain how values and norms developed, Sumner originated and elaborated his concepts of folkways and mores in his famous book *Folkways*, first published in 1907. The word means literally "the ways of the folk, the ways people have devised for satisfying their needs, for interacting with one another, and for conducting their lives."[15] Each society has different folkways, just as each has a different culture. Folkways, in brief, are customary ways of doing things in one's society. Mores, on the contrary, are former folkways judged to be essential to group wellbeing. The mores differ from folkways in the same way that moral conduct differs from merely customary conduct.

In brief, folkways which deal with societal welfare are mores. They are resistant to change for several reasons, primarily because they are deemed essential for the welfare and survival of the group. Mores are intergenerational obligations. One does not criticize them or reflect on them because one is born into a group with a reverence for them; they exert their influence before and after one is capable of reasoning. Such uncritical acceptance of the mores is particularly true of simple societies. Folkways can be changed more easily than mores; both can become institutionalized in the form of law.

Society-Culture-Personality and Gemeinschaft-Gesellschaft

Concepts that are often thought best expressed by the German words *Gemeinschaft* and *Gesellschaft* are important to be understood by the future dental health care professional who will be working in different types of societies and cultures. Since the terms represent extremes on a continuum, it would be difficult and inappropriate to attempt to classify a community as being purely *Gemeinschaft* or *Gesellschaft*. However, the fact that a community tends toward one or the other will affect both its perceptions and its acceptance of health care.

The community pole (*Gemeinschaft*) includes the simple, usually rural, social organization in which communication is direct and personal. At the societal pole (*Gesellschaft*) the relationships among individuals are impersonal and communication among them proceeds along channels determined by efficiency.

In attempting to effect any kind of dental health program, its advocates should attempt to understand *Gemeinschaft* (an essentially rural concept) and *Gesellschaft* (an essentially urban one). Such an understanding will help the future practitioner achieve more cooperation and acceptance in individuals from all levels of society, both young and old, rich and poor, white and nonwhite. If one wished to impress upon a community the need to use dental floss in addition to brushing, the approach in a *Gemeinschaft* community would be different from the approach in a *Gesellschaft* community. In a rural environment one would have to convince the persons in the community who control the power within the family. In a *Gesellschaft* one might get a good effect through television advertisements on children's programs.

Since people tend to move from rural to urban, or vice versa, there may be a tendency for an individual, group or society to develop a condition known as *anomie*—normlessness. In this situation, established common values and even common meanings are no longer understood or accepted; new meanings and contradictions are ever present. Some individuals involved in this kind of mobility may be referred to as "marginal." Louis Writh[16] used the term to refer to one whose self "is divided between the world that he has deserted and the world that will have none of him." Marginality is a concept that can be useful to the dental professional in understanding the patient undergoing role changes brought about by mobility. This concept can also be used as a starting point in a discussion of the treatment of neurotic and/or psychotic patients. This approach would lead to an investigation of a practitioner's role in dealing with the mentally ill patient.

On a national level, research has demonstrated the relationship between society, culture, personality and dental health care. For example, a study was done on youths in community dentistry in an Indian reservation. Results indicated that in addition to a myriad of other problems, the level of oral health and oral health education was even lower than that found in other socioeconomically depressed groups. The dental students who had participated in the project were able to grasp more fully the oral health problems confronting minority groups. The project operated a dental clinic for the Apache Indians in which students working with their own faculty and the dentists of the Indian Health Service provided both preventive and restorative services for ten weeks.[17]

Earlier studies have shown that if the Indian Health Service Dental Program was to continue in light of the rapid growth of the native population, the productivity of the existing dental staff would have to be increased. Thus, dental auxiliaries would have to perform expanded functions in a relatively short time.[18]

In 1973, a study described a program developed by the

University of Kentucky College of Dentistry. It was a five-year effort toward incremental dental care for school children in Wolfe County and in an economically depressed rural area of Appalachia. The dental treatment was provided by senior students who were required to participate in the program. The general objectives of the project included demonstrating the impact of community-wide programs of education and treatment on the attitudes of children and their parents toward dental care and determining the dental care requirements of children in a depressed area when care is provided on an incremental basis.[19]

In recent times, great interest has been placed on community care of the handicapped (for example, the blind, deaf, educationally subnormal, epileptic, maladjusted, physically handicapped, defective of speech, senile), who live in their homes. Results of a study have shown that this enthusiasm for community care must be welcomed only if the services that make it a reality can be provided. The handicapped and chronically sick do not primarily want sympathy and consolation; rather, they want help. Each health profession must, therefore, be responsive to the needs of these disadvantaged people and serve them with the same degree of attention it provides to the community at large. It is suggested that future developments in the health service to the community may eventually provide special regional facilities for the handicapped.

Another study pointed out that all phases of dentistry performed on the normal patient may be done on the hemophiliac with similar dental problems. Extreme care and meticulous skill will help prevent avoidable injury to soft tissue. Preventive dental care for hemophiliacs in the community should be taught and encouraged. Consultation with the patient's physician should precede any treatment, such cooperation allowing the hemophiliac to seek treatment with confidence.[20]

In 1974 a study was done on the effects of different communication techniques on the cooperation of the mentally retarded child undergoing dental work. There are over six million mentally retarded children in the United States and dental care for them constitutes a great problem, especially in terms of communication between the dentist and these children. Institutionalized mentally retarded subjects who initially were less cooperative appeared to benefit from some visual instruction prior to receiving dental treatment.[21]

From the standpoint of meeting dental needs of the aged in a society, the word "gerodontics" was coined. A study defines it as "that branch of dental service which is concerned with the effects of aging upon the occurrence, prevention, and treatment of dental disease." The author who postulated this concept of "gerodontics" asserted that he is concerned with the way dentists relate to this field and calls attention to the fact that all values of good oral health apply to the elderly with increasing significance in most cases. This is more so because the social and biological advantages of a healthy mouth are more needed and appreciated by the aged at a time in life when biological and sociological effectiveness is waning.[22]

In the past, additional studies from different cultures have clearly demonstrated the relationship between society-culture-personality and dental health care. For example, in 1971 it was reported that 45 percent of the West German population did not use a toothbrush. Thus, it was emphasized that any successful effort in dental health education ought to consider the enormous potential of the dentist in serving as a source of information and guidance.[23]

In England, it was noted that an understanding of personality was an essential factor in the assistance of apprehensive patients of any age through the more stressful aspects of dental treatment. Children have several ways of showing that they are anxious. They may cry, refuse to accept the simplest treatment or become babyish. The environment and atmosphere in which treatment is carried out is under the dentist's control. Stress is reduced by an approach that is sympathetic, understanding, unhurried, free of pain and within the realm of tolerance. The dentist's voice must be calm, friendly and confident, never harsh, domineering, teasing or critical. In brief, successful treatment will depend upon the patient's personality, the dentist's personality and the latter's understanding of the psychological factors involved.[24]

In 1970, research done in France concluded that several factors such as the relationship between the patient and the dentist and the age and sex of the patient are important in dental care. Fear is a significant aspect of dental treatment; manifestations of it are sweating, pallor, tremor and crying and mental resentment of the dentist. Psychological and sociological reasons are associated with such fear. The dentist's personality could play an important role in alleviating such fears.[25]

An investigation was conducted in Sweden to analyze and compare the environments of children with high caries frequency and children with low caries frequency. The families of these children were stratified into four social groups, as judged by income and education. More children with high caries incidence were found in group 4, the lowest socially; groups 1 and 2 had the lowest caries frequency. The social habits, attitudes and socioeconmic backgrounds of the families were found to be essential factors in the development of caries.[26]

In Poland, a study noted that preventive measures against oral diseases were necessary. It was suggested that mass prevention of caries should focus on the education of the population to mantain high oral hygiene standards. Clinics should instruct the public with films, talks and brochures. Water fluoridation ought to be correlated with caries prevalence. In brief, preventive dental care must be made available to the society at large.[27]

In the following chapter, attention will be given to the institution of the family—the most basic socializing agency and the unit of health and illness.

Chapter 2

The Family

This chapter deals with the problem of dental care from the perspective of the family. We will attempt to introduce some theories and research findings about the family in relation to health care. Health is defined, in Dubos' terms of adaptation, as the success of the organism in its efforts to respond adaptively to environmental challenges.[1] The definition with the widest agreement was proposed over thirty years ago by the World Health Organization of the United Nations in 1945. Here health is defined positively as a "state of complete physical, mental, and social well-being" and not as merely the absence of disease or infirmity. Thus, health is not an isolated phenomenon but rather is the result of the interaction of a complex variety of biological, geographic, psychological, social, and cultural factors.

The family, on the other hand, is the most permanent of all social institutions. It is the most fundamental agency for the socialization of the individual. There is no human society in which some form of the family does not exist.

It has been asserted that "the family is the unit of medical care because it is the unit of living."[2] Most obviously the family is related to health by the fact of biological inheritance of some diseases, such as sickle cell anemia, RH incompatibility, tendencies to diabetes, tuberculosis, and poor dentition. Heredity is responsible for darker teeth with translucent appearance. These darker teeth lose their enamel more readily than normal teeth and wear down more often to the gum line.[3]

Briefly, the functions of the family are sexual regulation, reproduction, the socialization of children, serving as a, or the, source of affection for its members, defining the status of children, and providing protection and security of the physical, economic, and psychological kinds. One disputed function of the family is the socialization of its members into the society. In general, the term socialization is used to describe the ways in which individuals learn the values, beliefs and roles that underwrite the social system in which they participate.

The sick role, developed in the socialization process, is most important in physical and mental disorders. A patient acts out his sick role in relation to his physician, his dentist, his family and other members of society in the manner in which he has internalized this role from infancy. According to Parsons,[4] there are four aspects to the sick role of patients. These are that sick persons are exempted from their normal responsibilities, depending upon the seriousness of their illness; that sick persons cannot help themselves and must be cared for by others; that the sick role is viewed as a misfortune, hence it is assumed that the sick person will want to get well, and is under an actual obligation to do so; and finally, that it is the obligation of the sick person to seek competent help, usually from a physician or dentist, and to cooperate with the professional in getting well. As previously mentioned, the classic study of the way family and culture socialize an individual to the sick role is Mark Zborowski's on the cultural components of pain.

In general, the behaviors and attitudes of sick persons are formed during the socialization process within the family by the parent's response to the child's crying. Normally a child's crying is responded to by sympathy and concern on the part of the parents. However, by an overprotective and worried attitude concerning the crying, parents foster complaints and tears. From this a child may learn to pay too much attention to the potentially painful aspects of experiences and to look for sympathy and help too often. The family, through the socialization process, influences the individual's definition of health care.

Family roles can be seriously affected by illness, bringing about a reshaping of roles and role responsibilities. Role reversal between parents is a common one, in which the breadwinner's responsibility is switched, and patterns of child care may need to change. For example, if a longshoreman loses his leg through an on-the-job accident, he will no longer be able to act out his occupational role (since the use of both legs would be necessary for him to perform his work successfully). His wife may now become the breadwinner and he becomes the homemaker. These transitions can be sources of confusion in identity for children during the early developmental stages especially if there has been prior inadequate role performance on the part of the parents toward their children.

The family also influences health care through its *nurturing* of the individual. A family of ten crowded into an inadequate home without sufficient heat and enough finances for balanced meals will be more likely to become ill, and the individual's view of health will reflect his or her experiences under such living conditions.

Members of a family share hereditary characteristics, a common environment, and common modes of thought and behavior. These factors to a large degree are responsible for a family's susceptibilty to disease. The rate of infection will spread depending upon the family's material and social environment.[5]

The idea of family has a deep root in us all and directs many of our actions, although we may not realize it consciously. It directs the ways we perceive health and illness, and the things we expect from medical and dental health care. The education and income earned by a family are associated with the dental health of members of the family. For example, the higher the income of a family the less is the likelihood that young members would have periodontal disease.[6] One study published in 1974 showed that families with incomes of less than $3000 had an incidence of periodontal disease as high as 49 percent in youths aged 12 to 17 years; for families with an income of over $10,000, the incidence drops to 21 percent. Also, the education of parents is closely associated with periodontal disease of adolescents. The Periodontal Index decreased from a high of 0.61 for those whose parents had five years or less of education to 0.16 for those whose parents had 17 years or more.[7] Further, as income and education increase in a family unit, the average number of decayed and missing teeth decreases. By contrast, decayed and missing teeth increase for families who prior to 1974 were earning less than three thousand dollars.[8]

Recent research has demonstrated that the degree of oral

cleanliness among youths of all races varied according to annual family income. Thus, adolescents in the lower income groups had appreciably poorer oral hygiene than those in the higher income groups.[9]

Given the role of the family in relation to health care we will turn our attention now to various research findings on the family and some selected sociological concepts and theories which will be helpful in understanding the interdependence of these two institutions in society.

Development of the Self

In order to appreciate more fully how attitudes and values are developed toward health and illness, we should explain the development of the *self* and the *self concept*. The self concept involves the assumption that personalities act according to the way they perceive themselves (their self concept) and according to the way they perceive the social situation. A social situation by definition would include all forces acting upon the individual at any given moment in time.

There are two general ways in which we can examine the origins of the self and the self concept. The first is egocentric; it suggests that human beings innately know that they are distinct and separate and it implies that the self is relatively complete before it comes into contact with anyone or anything else. The second view posits that man develops his self and self concept through interaction with the world. Charles Horton Cooley viewed this process as a development of the "looking-glass self"—in which self definitions are based upon the response of other individuals. In the "looking-glass self" people develop their feelings about themselves in response to the way other people treat them. They come to learn how other people view them and this affects their view of themselves. This is also the basis of George Herbert Mead's theory of *play, game*, and the *generalized other*.

Mead based his research on that of Cooley, who asserted the interdependence of self and society. Mead, on the other hand, noted that the individual internalizes the role behavior of others during the socialization process. For Mead, the "I" is a person as an actor. The "Me" or the "self" is a person's perception of what other people think about him or her. Individuals have to develop a coherent "self" out of the many different ways they are treated by the different people with whom they interact. Thus, the "I" and the "Me" are constantly working together to form a person's personality.

The self develops through the processes of social experiences and activities. But almost all social exchanges between human beings involve language, either spoken or written. This is one principal form of communication, and it is only through communication that we can learn about the perspectives of others. Therefore, it is essential for the development of the self that one learns the common symbols of the language of one's group. The most important agent for the socialization of the child—which, of course includes teaching the child to speak—is the family.

There are other ways in which the family contributes to this growth. Mead proposes two major steps of development—play and game. In *play*, the child assumes one role which he or she has seen enacted by some other individual. These roles may follow in rapid sucession; one time the child will play mother, then the same child will play father or teacher, or any other role with which there has been contact. Most often, however, the children will take on the roles of the significant others in their lives. These are the people whom the child values greatly, and the greater the value of the other individual, the more important the role. The child "plays-at-the-role" and attempts to identify with the role being played.

The second stage, *game*, finds the individual taking on the perspective of all others involved in some common activity. Games always have some sort of rules, whether they are explicit, as in the football field, or implicit, as in daily interactions with the next-door neighbors. The essential element of this stage is that the individual feels a unity with the other selves in the interaction; they are called the *generalized others*.

The attitude and perspective of the *generalized other* is the attitude and perspective of the group as a whole. Individuals internalize this and govern their conduct accordingly—they play-the-role expected of them. In this way, the community exercises control over the conduct of its members and influences their decisions.

In brief, for Mead, knowing one's role in society includes knowing all the roles that bear upon it. For example, the patient's role is defined in relationship to that of the dentist. The student's role is defined in terms of that of the teacher. Thus, a child might learn many adults roles without ever actually practicing them. This knowledge is available to the child, should he or she be placed in an environment where they are called on to play one of these roles. Children know these roles only if they see them, and might learn them inadequately.

The "Self" and Dental Care Research

The development, therefore, of the *self concept* according to Cooley and Mead is most important in the delivery of dental health care. Brooks and Bagramian[10] asserted that the two goals of the project Head Start in Washtenaw County, Michigan, were to provide the most complete dental care for the largest number of children and to provide dental education for families—both children and parents. Dental education included tooth brushing instructions and introducing the child to the dentist to allay fright.

In 1973, Douglas and Stacey[11] reviewed, in part, a study by Lambert and Freeman entitled "The Clinic Habit." This was an extensive study of dental health which the reviewers claimed to be a "unique combination of the analytic skill of social scientists and the health expertise of dental public health." Lambert and Freeman studied all Brookline families with at least one child 17 or under who was in a public or parochial high school in the 1964 academic year. The families were ranked by occupational status and oral examinations were performed on the children.

The reviewers felt that Lambert and Freeman were able to demonstrate convincingly that patients' dental conditions are related to their dental behavior. Dental behavior in turn is linked strongly to the practices of dental and medical health of the entire family.

A recent study of parents as behavior modifiers showed some interesting results; these would be applied to dental care for those wishing to train young children in good oral hygiene habits or to help modify the poor habits of older children. The study[12] involved welfare and middle-class parents in Madison, Wisconsin. The purpose was to modify the problem behaviors in their children. The findings indicated that welfare parents who were put together with middle-class parents for training were better motivated than those who were segregated. Further, the study noted that unless contradictory data appear, one can conclude that homogeneity in group structure is not a desirable condition in programs of social education for welfare parents.

The kinds of foods eaten by children during their socialization process may have a direct relationship to the health of their teeth. For example, among families living on unsophisticated diets, as in many parts of Africa, tooth decay is absent or rare, yet it becomes common with urbanization and change of diet. Rural school children on the island of Lewis, Scotland, had excellent teeth. Alterations in diet, however, resulted in an increase in caries. By adolescence, more than a third of the school children's teeth were decayed. Among the reasons suggested for the deterioration of the children's teeth was increased intake of refined carbohydrate foods, particularly sugar. The study indicated that one must devise ways to retain or to alter the dietary habits of people for good oral health.[13]

Structure of the Family

Every social institution has some sort of structure or framework which helps to put the needs or purposes of the institution into the world of action, so that it can serve the interests of society and the members who compose it. The family as a social institution has its framework or structure within which it can carry out the purposes for which it exists. Most individuals are members of two families during their lives. The first is the family of origin, in which our earliest experiences take place. The second is the family of *marriage*, in which we enact the role of parents. It is within the network of familial relationships that we develop our attitudes and values toward health and illness. Attitudes are tendencies to feel and act in certain ways. Values, on the other hand, are measures of desirability.

The family, as we have noted earlier, is the most universal of all human institutions. It varies widely in structure from the consanguine type (*i.e.*, extended kin groups which include a wide variety of related persons) to conjugal families consisting simply of an adult pair (male and female) and their children. The conjugal family acts as a source of "refuge" in mass society—a place where the individual may engage in genuinely personal relationships in a world which is largely impersonal—and is primarily found in developed societies such as the United States and Europe. The consanguine family, based upon the group relationship of a large number of people, is found chiefly in developing nations such as India.

In the past, many authors have given us a description of different types of families. P.A. Sorokin,[14] for example, presents three types, the *compulsive*, the *contractual*, and the *familistic*. In the compulsive family, the bond holding members together is not love but force and the relationship is based on exploitation, cruelty and deprivation. The contractual type brings profit and advancement to the particpants but is devoid of love (or hatred). The familistic type is based on mutual love between the spouses and is characterized by devotion and sacrifice, solidarity, sharing, permanence and stability. Sorokin feels that the three types of families have been present in all societies, changing in proportion with time; the type most prevalent in today's Western society is thought by Sorokin to be contractual.

The type of family a person comes from can help us understand the behavior of the patient and members of the family toward the sick person. For example, in severe coronary cases, increasing demands are made on the family to adjust their customary routines to the patient's needs. One can expect, therefore, that if the family type was close (familistic), each member concerned about the others prior to the illness, then there would be a greater willingness for members of the family to adjust their roles to help the sick person. On the contrary, if the family type was contractual and/or compulsive, then the family members would be less willing to make the sacrifices to aid the sick individual.

Another term for describing a type of family is the "empty shell," first used by William J. Goode.[15] In this kind of family there are no primary group ties such as concern, love and security for the members. Communication and sharing are at the minimum, so solidarity and permanence are undermined. Each member of this type of family is self-seeking; there is very little respect or even recognition of the needs of the other members. As a result, divorce and juvenile delinquency are frequent, especially in a large urban society. The offspring tend to leave the home of their parents as soon as they can make their own way in society. This type of family is one which has forfeited all of its functions (except the reproductive) and has, therefore, lost control over its members. The "empty shell family" has been known by various other names. It is like P.A. Sorokin's "contractual family"; Zimmerman and Cervantes spoke of the same sort of family as an "atomistic" one that rejects traditional and religious values and provides an unstable environment for the socialization of children.

The way stress is handled within a family during a sudden crisis will depend upon the type of familial relationships prior to the episode. For example, stress within a family may lead to infectious illness. Research done at the Family Medicine Unit at Harvard Medical School has demonstrated that "common crises such as death of grandparents, a change of residence, a loss of a father's job, and a child's being subjected to unusual pressure occur four times more frequently in the two weeks period prior to the appearance of streptococcal infections than in the two weeks afterward."[16]

Another kind of crisis in which the type of family plays an important role is the biological inheritance factor. If people learn that they are carriers of diseases which affect their children, or learn that they are the recipient of such familiar diseases, complicated emotional problems in family interaction can result. For example, the birth of a deformed infant may be accompanied by a guilt reaction on the part of both parents. One can speculate upon the emotional disturbances of the family in the specific case of muscular dystrophy which is carried by the female and attacks the male. The need of a parent to deny knowledge about such discomforting facts is understandable; however, there is a tendency for the parent to believe the facts must be disproved and to seek continuously other advice in order to get different answers. At this stage of the crisis, there is a great need to see the family as a unit of treatment. Whether or not the family is viewed as such will depend partially upon the type of familial relationships prior to the episode.[17,18]

Family stucture can also be examined from the standpoint of the utilization of dental health care. Studies reported by Odin W. Anderson[19] indicated that "16 percent of the families in 1964 accounted for three-fourths of the total expenditures"; 6 percent accounted for one-half, while "2 percent of the families accounted for one-fourth of the total expenditures." For individuals, in contrast to the family, "59 percent had no dental expenditures and only 9 percent had expenditures of fifty dollars or more. The mean expenditure for all individuals was 18 dollars.

"Similar patterns exist for dental visits. The mean number of visits per family was 4.6. Furthermore, 3 percent of the families accounted for one-fourth of the visits and 26 percent of the families accounted for three-fourths of the visits. For individuals, in contrast to the family, 55 percent of the sample made no visits to the dentist. The mean number of visits for all persons was 1.5."[20]

Thus far, we have seen that the structure and functions of the family play a very important role in the lives of individuals who are confronted with decisions of health and illness. The family, as noted previously, is the unit of health care because it is the unit of living. This concept—the unit of health care—is a broad one, encompassing mental and dental as well as general health care. Thus, it is important for us to be aware of the various types of family therapy so that a dental practitioner may have a better understanding of how to deal with a patient who is undergoing treatment.

Forms of Family Therapy

While many families function with little assistance from outside agencies, an increasing number have sought professional help to make their family situation more livable. "Family counseling" has been viewed as the most logical solution for family problems and yet, this counseling does not follow a set pattern. The type of counseling rendered is dependent on both the family situation and the orientation of the therapist. All forms of family therapy view the family as an integrated unit comprised of individuals. While some forms of therapy place emphasis on the concept of integrated *unit*, other forms emphasize the *individual* within the unit.

Although each form of therapy views the family as a viable unit of treatment, certain "schools" conceive of the family in different terms. The entire picture of family therapy might be viewed as a continuum, with individual orientation and group orientation constituting the end points.

The three approaches are ideal types of family therapy. The psychoanalytic school emphasizes the individual rather than the group. Some key concepts are: *psychic determinism*, which states that each event in an individual's life stems from specific conscious or unconscious causes—nothing happens by chance; *the unconscious mental life*: it is assumed that both therapist and patient will develop insight from each other unconsciously, before the patient's emotional problems are resolved; and *genetic orientation*, in which mental phenomena are the product of the interplay between the environment and a biological organism whose development is largely predetermined.

At the opposite end of the family therapy continuum is the communicative-interactive approach. This approach places primary importance on the family unit and de-emphasizes individual family members. Since this form of therapy centers on family communication, the key concept focuses on this process. The *double-bind* concept, grounded in the belief that communication is the chief factor in human interaction, states that a single communication presents a number of messages (conveyed both verbally and nonverbally), for example, a parent's verbal message saying "grow up" and nonverbal actions which tell the child that he is still a "baby." Since communication is a process between individuals, this form of therapy necessitates more than one person's being involved in the therapy sessions.

Family homeostasis is another concept crucial to the communicative-interactive approach. The family operates within a certain set framework, and this framework might include the presence of a sick family member. Although a cure might be beneficial to the individual member, it might serve to throw the family homeostasis out of balance (for example, the family does not know how to cope with a "well" member). In attempting to preserve the status quo, the family might continue to view the individual as "sick" or might view another family member as "sick" in an attempt to replace the formerly "sick" component—a factor viewed as necessary for the family's survival.

The final approach examined, the integrative approach, focuses on the integration of aspects of the psychoanalytic and the communicative-interactive. In general, this mode of treatment is an eclectic attempt to include both the individual and the family unit in therapy. Since it examines both concepts, it is in fact a study of the individual in his or her environment; the key concept in the approach is role. Role is viewed as a pattern of acts, partially determined by culture, and carried out in a social situation; a role does not exist in isolation, but is determined by the reciprocal role of a role partner. The family is viewed as a system in which roles are learned and then acted out by its members.

Role complementarity exists when individuals and their role partners have mutual perceptions of their roles. When mutual perceptions, however, do not exist, role conflict occurs and equilibrium breaks down. Since the family system is comprised of three subsystems—the marital relationship, the parent-child relationship and the sibling relationship—and these subsystems are interrelated, role conflict in one subsystem will extend to the other subsystems.

In brief, therefore, although family might take a number of approaches and employ a variety of techniques, all forms recognize the individual as a member of a family unit, which to varying degrees, determines his or her personality as well as relationship to the environment.

The Changing American Family

Since the American Revolution there has been a decrease

in the size of family units. Then the average completed family size was 5.7 persons. At present, the average size is between three and four members. This decrease is the result of an increasingly literate and industrialized society. New family patterns have also resulted from the general acceptance of divorce. Over the past fifty years the divorce rate in the United States has probably doubled. In the 1970's in many legal jurisdictions about one of every two marriages was ending in divorce.

The increase in women's employment, a result of a more industrialized society, has brought drastic changes in American family life. It has changed the labor and authority patterns of the family. Outside agencies have replaced parental functions, and authority patterns have become more equalitarian.

Changes in the structure of the American family have resulted in new functional changes. Although the two primary functions of procreation and child-rearing remain the same, there has been an increased recognition of the socialization process, increased responsibility to render affection and companionship, and a movement from economic production to economic consumption of the members of the family unit.

Irrespective of the changes that may occur in the family in future years, it will provide the basis on which each person can develop his or her own humanity. Without this, humankind will become merely another machine furthering the cause of technology. Thus, in contributing to the growth of the individual's personality, the family, as a primary group, will continue to foster the patterns of society and culture.

There has been, and there will be, many experiments in family living, some of which will fail. But the institution of the family as a primary group and as the basic unit of society will not fail. The present definition of the family may be expanded, as it is reformed to meet the needs of persons in our rapidly changing society. Whatever changes may occur, the family will be the fundamental institution for the delivery of health care. As such, it will be the unit of dental care as well.

Chapter 3

Social Class

Stratification and Society

In all societies individuals tend to become arranged in some sort of hierarchy in every stratum of which the members possess certain characteristics in common, which serve also to separate them from members of other strata. Some people are more highly valued than others. There might be several classses in a society and they would lie one above the other. Hence, the system is usually described as a system of social stratification. Stratification, therefore, refers to the division of society into higher and lower economic classes and prestige groups. It is a continuum in which every person has a position; the position, in turn, provides the basis for according certain rights and privileges.

Social stratification is an integral part of the interlocking system of society-culture-personality. By definition, a social system is a patterned relationship of roles. We have previously asserted that a role is a pattern of expected behavior related to a certain position within a society. A role, therefore, is related to the concept of status which is, in the simplest terms, an individual's position in society. For example, a dental auxiliary activates his or her status in a dental clinic, performing a role in relation to patients, dentists and other allied workers.

There are three types of statuses: achieved, assumed, and ascribed. Achieved status is that which individuals attain as a result of their own efforts. Assumed status is obtained by means of various contacts such as business, social, or professional rather than by an individual's own effort. Ascribed status is derived from attributes over which the individual has no control such as age, sex, race and nationality. Ascribed status normally cannot be changed. These three statuses are closely related to the concepts of caste and class in either a *Gemeinschaft* or *Gesellschaft* society.

A class, by definition, consists of a stratum of people of similar social rank. The individuals have approximately equal positions in society which may be achieved or may be ascribed. They have some opportunity for movement upward or downward to another class. A society which is based on a class structure is called an "open society." A system is open if individuals can move from stratum to stratum—*i.e.*, every status can be achieved.

A woman's status can more easily than a man's be altered in either direction, because she shares her husband's status. Western males do not ordinarily directly gain in status through marriage; however, "marrying money" may bring status elevation in the future. By marrying into an influential family a man or woman may obtain the "connections" necessary to assume positions otherwise unobtainable. Status can be altered also by achievements and failures—by achievement is understood an extraordinary, usually unexpected performance which calls wider public attention to the abilities of a person. Not all achievements result in social mobility, but a poor person who acquires wealth or an unknown writer who wins a literary prize will experience an improvement in status. Only remarkable achievements will affect status. As a rule only top performances cause upward mobility; failure and misdeeds similarly affect downward mobility largely through their scale. Further ideas on status can be found in Bergel's *Social Stratification.*[1]

A caste, on the other hand, is a social group into which a person is born and from which he or she finds it very difficult to escape. Social position in the caste is ascribed rather than achieved. A caste system prevents the individual from achieving higher status or social position than was ascribed at birth. The classical example of a caste system is found in India, where individuals are born into castes which determine their social status for life. A society with a caste system is often referred to as a "closed society."

The concepts of class and caste are, in turn, associated with mobility and/or immobility. Social mobility is one way of classifying the wide range of stratification systems in societies. It is the rise and fall of the individual in group positions. It is the movement of people from one stratum of society to another. Social mobility refers specifically to vertical mobility, which is movement upward or downward on the social scale. For example, a hygienist upon graduation may move from a working class to a middle class position. Physical or geographical mobility, on the other hand, refers to movement from one place of residence to another. For example, a family may move from one poverty area to another poverty area. This type of mobility is not necessarily related to social mobility, even though in practice the two are frequently correlated. Closely related to physical or geographical mobility is the shift in one's occupation without a corresponding change in one's status. Two basic kinds of mobility can be distinguished: the intra-generational—the extent to which persons change their status during their own life—and the inter-generational—the extent to which an individual's status differs from that of his or her parents or grandparents.

The ingredients which are necessary for social mobility are ability, ambition and sponsorship. However, even though individuals may be able to possess these ingredients, they can be confronted with several problems. For example, they would have to make a role adjustment to their new position. They would have to unlearn old and relearn new skills required as upward mobility brings new duties and obligations. Problems may arise due to the disruption of primary group relations. An individual who has changed social class may discover that he or she now has very little in common with family and friends. This discovery often leads to loneliness and disillusionment.

In the process of social mobility, there is usually a deferred gratification pattern. The postponement of present satisfactions to achieve later goals is rather typical of persons in the middle class. These individuals aspire for upper-class status and in the process encounter fears of returning to a lower-class position in society. They encounter marginality in which they are caught between two worlds—the upper-class and the lower-class—and they seem to belong to neither group. The marginality affecting such persons could lead to anomie, that is, a general alienation or lack of norms. This in turn can lead to severe mental illness.

Since it is possible in the United States to change status during an individual's lifetime, the distinctions between the classes are not clearly defined. W. Lloyd Warner in his detailed research of social stratification in representative communities throughout the United States divided Americans into six social classes. These classes were subdivisions of the classic upper, middle, and lower classes. In Warner's six-class typology over half the population falls into the lower classes. Each class above the upper-lower class in the hierarchy is smaller than the preceding one. The middle class is expanding as the society grows more technical.

August B. Hollingshead of Yale University presented five social classes in his important work, *Elmtown's Youth.* He later utilized the same five social classes with Frederick C. Redlich in their now classic study, *Social Class and Mental Illness.* Hollingshead's five social classes are:

I. Upper (U)—This class includes wealthy families whose heads are business or professional leaders in the community;

II. Upper Middle (UM)—College graduates in high managerial positions or in the lesser ranking professions; well-to-do but with no substantial wealth;

III. Lower Middle (LM)—Small proprietors, white collar workers, salesmen and skilled manual workers;

IV. Upper Lower (UL)—Predominantly semiskilled factory workers with no more than high school education;

V. Lower Lower (LL)—Mostly semiskilled factory hands and unskilled laborers; many of the individuals have not completed elementary grades.

Although there are many indicators which influence the prestige judgments Americans make about groups, the following categories offer a general overview of social class indicators:

income and/or wealth (amounts and from what source derived)

education (levels and type of school attended)

occupation or profession (personal accomplishments/skills)

family background (social class origins, patterns of socialization)

authority and power (economic, political, professional)

prestige (how well known and highly regarded members of this group or occupation are)

service to the community (how much benefit to the community the group or occupation contributes)

personal characteristics (charisma, character, reputation, intelligence, beauty, popularity, etc.)

In addition to Hollingshead's "Two-Factor Index of Social Position," Warner developed the "Index of Status Characteristics," while Chapin formulated the "living room scale." The Warner system consisted of a weighted scoring of the four factors of social class: occupation, source of income, house type, and dwelling area; Chapin, on the other hand, assigned a score value to the quality and type of furnishings found in the family living room. In both cases, the goal is to come up with a numerical score which can then be ranked along with the score obtained for other subjects in the study (or, perhaps, against a standardized range presumably prevailing for the whole society). The most essential values or attitudes which shape the behavior of the majority of each social class are depicted.

There are three approaches to the analysis of the social strata in which people are placed: objective, subjective and reputational. In the objective approach, the main focus is directed to indices such as occupation, education, place of residence or the power a person possesses. In the subjective approach, people are asked to classify themselves into a particular social class. For example, individuals would be asked the question: "If you had to say what social class you belong to, which would it be?" The reputational approach is obtained by asking informants to classify other people.

Thus, people's social class position become a way of life for them. It influences their pattern of attitudes and values, their religious views, their informal modes of behavior, the kinds of health care treatment they receive, and their utilization of dental care.

Class Distinctions and Dental Care

It is helpful for dental health care workers to be aware of a patient's social class. Koos,[2] for example, asserts that upper-class persons are more likely than lower-class persons to view themselves as ill when they are aware of particular symptoms. When questioned about specific symptoms, they reported more frequently than lower-class persons that they seek a doctor's advice.

Indeed, socioeconomic status is clearly associated with certain kinds of diesases. Since oral health is a part of general health and hence affects the total well-being of individuals, it is important that we examine briefly other diseases in relation to one's class position in society. Research studies in Great Britain, for example, suggest that mortality rates in general, but especially infant and neonatal mortality rates, increased as class position decreased. Morbidity rates for certain diseases, mostly infectious and parasitic ones associated with poverty, follow the same pattern.[3]

Susser and Watson[4] suggest that gastroenteritis among infants, and bronchitis, pneumonia and tuberculosis are major causes of deaths in social classes IV and V (the two lowest social classes), while mortality rates of these diseases are much lower in classes I and II. On the other hand, some diseases are apparently more common—that is, are diagnosed more frequently—among the wealthy classes. These include coronary heart disease, poliomyelitis, leukemia and cirrhosis of the liver. For the most part, differences in mortality rates can be ascribed to class-linked social environment factors as well as to differences in occupation and lifestyles.

Chronic disease rates are greater in poor families—those in lower socioeconomic classes—than in comfortable and well-to-do families. The majority of the poor in the South, Southwest, Florida and Appalachia have no health or hospital insurance to provide health care. A 1971 study found that, as a result, 29 percent of the families had chronic illnesses if the income was less than $2000, as compared to 7.5 percent if the family had an annual income of $7000 or more (the dollar figures were significantly higher of course by the late 1970's). Persons in this study whose family income was less than $2000 had double the number of days of restricted activity in comparison with families who earned $7000. Lower income families have more multiple hospital episodes than higher income families. In the 1971 study children under 15 years of age averaged two visits to a physician per year in a family whose annual income was under $2000, compared to 4.4 visits for children whose family income was at least $7000. The hospital stay for the poor is longer and their mortality is higher.[5]

In recent years, however, many major American universities have begun to involve themselves in the quality of medical and dental care for the people in lower socioeconomic classes—the poor and disadvantaged citizens of the country. Howard University, with its theme, "If I Can Help Somebody," took steps to help relieve the health care needs of the people of Quitman County, Mississippi.[6] The objective of the project was to develop a three-part program in medicine, dentistry, and community development which would establish a comprehensive approach to improve health services, and, in turn, enhance the overall quality of life in Quitman County. A student survey found that the average person had not visited a dentist within five years. A dental component was included in the overall health care program. It consisted of a dental clinic for oral rehabilitation, a program in preventive dentistry and a program to train dental aides.

In Contra Costa County, California, a study of nearly 4000 five-year-old children showed that the prevalence of dental caries was inversely related to socioeconomic status.[7] Children in the lowest socioeconomic group had 60 percent more carious teeth (decayed teeth diagnosed for extraction, and filled teeth) than those in the highest group, while a much lower proportion of the former were free of caries altogether. Similar results were found in a survey of school children in Buffalo, New York.[8]

In North Carolina, a research project was done to study the caries experience of white and nonwhite children, at ages 6 through 11 and of differing socioeconomic classes, in fluoridated and nonfluoridated communities.[9] In the nonfluoridated community, the white children of upper socioeconomic status had a much lower dental caries rate than children of either race in the low socioeconomic group. In the fluoridated area, there were only minor differences in the permanent teeth of all groups; among the primary teeth, however, the caries rate for the upper socioeconomic groups was better than for the others.

Koos in *The Health of Regionville*[10] identified some of the factors which influence the attitude of individuals toward dental treatment. The population was divided into three socioeconomic groups, namely, Class I, which included business and professional persons; Class II, consisting of skilled and semiskilled workers; and Class III, made up of unskilled workers. Almost 95 percent of the Class I families indicated that they had a family dentist, in contrast to 12.5 percent of households in Class III. The reason submitted for visiting a dentist varied significantly among the three classes. Fifty percent of the respondents in Class III and 9 percent of the subjects in Class II reported that they went to dentists only to have a tooth extracted. On the contrary, however, 52 percent of the individuals in Class I indicated that prophylaxis and examination were the reasons for seeking dental care. Only 14 percent of the respondents in Class III listed these preventive services as the reason for visiting a dentist.[11]

These attitudes toward dental health care are somewhat similar to lower socioeconomic classes in other cultures. For example, during the colonial years in Guyana, South America, many people who lived in the villages and estates did not visit a dentist even for an extraction. They allowed the tooth to decay and as it became gradually more painful they would go to the local drug dispenser (a person who had no formal training in dentistry) to have the tooth pulled. The dispenser, who was called "Doc," would have a long line of patients, some with swollen jaws, waiting in his drug store, at the back of which he possessed a few dental instruments for use in extractions. He called each patient loudly and placed a tincture of iodine on the diseased tooth, warning the patient not to move. At that time fear engulfed the patient strongly, and in many instances the person would be screaming long before an instrument was placed in the mouth. The screaming was heard by the other patients awaiting their turn to be treated. Fear permeated the atmosphere and patients would return home only to be told by members of the family that they had to return to the "doctor." As the tooth was pulled from the patients who were brave enough to undergo the ordeal, they were given glasses of salt water to rinse their mouths in the yard. The dispenser received a quarter or so from the patient, who was sent home.

In the United States, research has demonstrated the association of filled teeth with increasing income and decayed or extracted teeth with decreasing income. The relationship of dental health of American youths with their family income was investigated in one study; figures indicate that numbers of filled teeth steadily rise with the family's income, from 1.6 in youths whose families earned less than $3000 (as of 1974) to 5.4 teeth in those whose families earned $15,000 or more. Numbers of decayed or missing teeth showed a decrease corresponding to an increase in the family's income: children of families earning less than $3000 averaged 3.9 decayed or missing teeth, compared to only one tooth for those of families earning $15,000 or more.[12]

The frequency with which orthodontic treatment was sought bore a striking relation to family income. For example, a study done in 1971 showed that the percentage of visits involving orthodontic treatment ranged from a low of 14 for children whose families earned lesss than $7000 yearly to a high of 38.1 for those whose families earned $15,000 or more. Similar findings were made for youths and young adults.[13]

A relationship was also found between the oral hygiene status of children in the United States and the amount of yearly income earned by their families. As family income increased, the

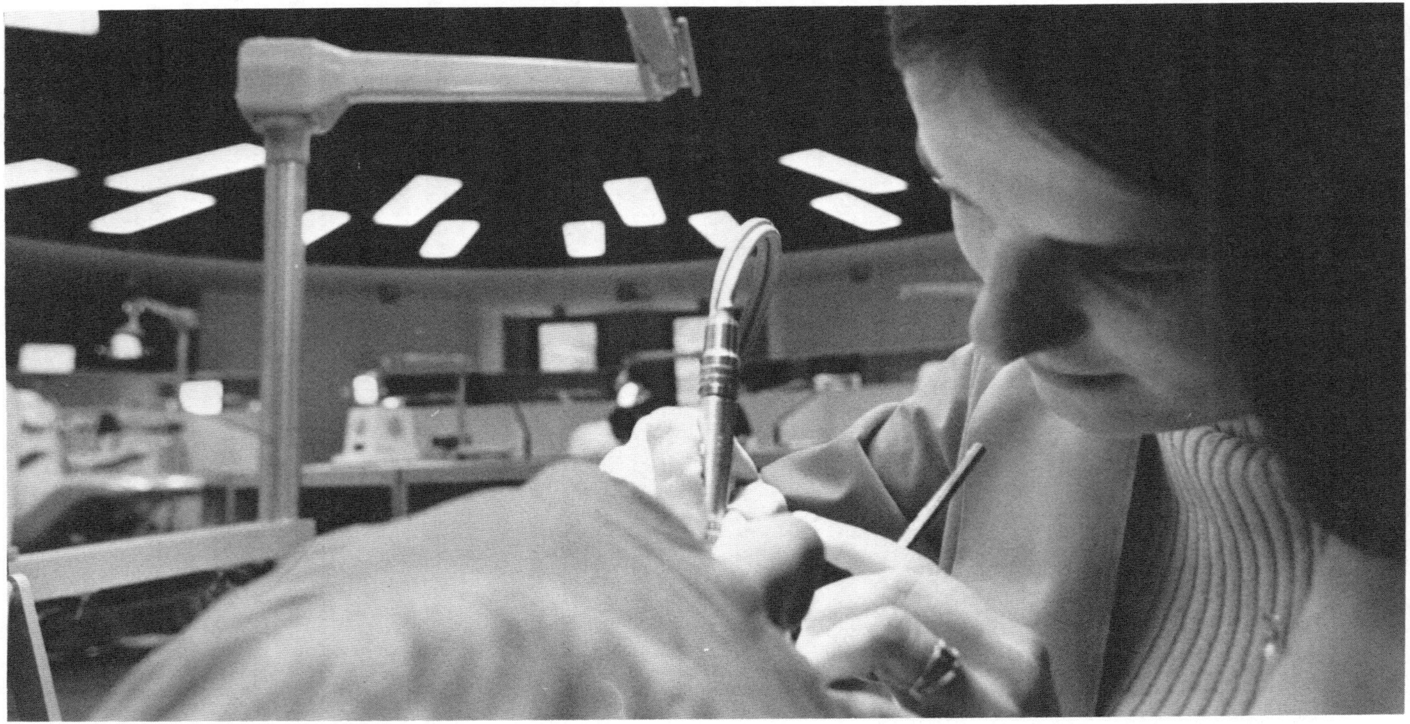

Hygienist performing dental prophylaxis (photograph by Ralph R. Lobene)

average scores of the OHI-S (simplified Oral Hygiene Index) per child decreased. The decrease in the OHI-S was consistent, with progressively smaller mean scores occurring with each added increment of income. Thus, in early 1970's income terms, the index fell from a high of 1.69 for children in families earning less than $3000 to 1.31 for those with family incomes of $7000 to $9999 and, finally, to a low of 1.21 for those in the highest income group.[14]

We have noted previously in this chapter that income and education are indices of socioeconomic status. Studies have shown that there are associations between toothless persons and their income and education. For example, as family income increases, the percentage of persons who had lost all their natural teeth decreases. The percentage of those 65 and over who had lost all their teeth varied from 58.5 percent of those in families earning less than $3000, to only 35.2 percent of those earning $15,000 or more.[15] In addition, the proportion of toothless, or edentulous, persons was related to the educational attainment of the individual: in each age group over 25, the percentage remained the same or decreased as educational level increased. Additional figures show the percentage of edentulous persons of family income and level of education for persons aged 45 to 64 years of age and older. "For each of the three income levels the percentage decreased as educational level increased. For each level of education the percentage decreased as the level of family income increased. In the age group 45-64, 36.9 percent of the persons with fewer than 9 years of education and a family income of less than $5,000 had lost all their natural teeth. In this same age group only 12.1 percent of the individuals with 12 or more years of education and family income of $10,000 or more were edentulous. Even for persons 65 or over, only three out of 10 individuals who had 12 or more years of education and a family income of $10,000 or more were edentulous."[16]

Research studies have shown that utilization of dental services is directly related to the education and occupational level of the head of the household.[17] Also, increases in family income are associated with corresponding increases in utilization. Further, a family's perceived ability to pay for dental services is indirectly related to utilization.[18]

Caries experience and levels of treatment vary significantly by socioeconomic status. A recent study has shown that children of low status had greater mean numbers of decayed surfaces at all ages compared with children of middle socioeconomic status. By age 5.5 years, children in the low status group had an average of about three additional decayed surfaces when compared with children in the middle status group.[19]

The above research further indicated that children in the low status group had an average of 13.9 percent of their decayed teeth treated by restoration or extraction in contrast to 23.9 percent in the middle classes. Also, children in the low socioeconomic classes at each level of age had greater percentages with caries experience and also greater average numbers of decayed teeth and surfaces. For five-year-old children in the middle class the average number of decayed teeth was 4.28 compared with an average of 6.26 for the children of low status. The children of the low socioeconomic group also had an average of about four additional decayed surfaces compared with children in the middle status group.[20]

In a dental survey in Texas, 1010 students aged five to 13 were randomly selected from 10 elementary schools to study the prevalence of dental caries and gingivitis. Data gathered included age, sex, ethnic status and socioeconomic level. Results showed that students of low socioeconomic backgrounds had the largest number of decayed teeth and the fewest number of filled teeth.[21]

In a study of a surburban Buffalo community with a population of 52,400, socioeconomic status and factors influencing the dental health practices of mothers were analyzed.[22] Findings showed that education, family income and father's occupation were most influential in defining social class. In addition, children's attitudes toward dental care followed from the mother's attitude toward tooth brushing frequency and number of dental visits. For each socioeconomic group, the key factor varied; members of the lower socioeconomic class were most influenced by level of parental education determined by tooth brushing frequency; for the middle socioeconomic group, education of the mother was the key factor. While the relationships in the upper socioeconomic class were similar to the other two, there were two significant differences: both social class and parental education had no effects on maternal practices.

A recent study has shown that there are significant relationships among socioeconomic status, loss of teeth, and participation in a dental project.[23] Socioeconomic status was scored on the basis of the father's occupation and the level of each parent's education. Among the findings of this study are that participation of parents in a dental examination was related significantly to the level of education of both sexes and the occupation of the father; that socioeconomic status, participation in a dental examination, loss of teeth in adults, and dental debris in their children were interrelated; and that participation in the study and loss of teeth reflect dental attitudes and behavior which were related to educational level.

Over the past years, studies have demonstrated the need to educate the lower classes to the benefits of specific health innovations and good health prerequisites in general. Research has shown that "the health educator must recognize and take account of the norms and standards of the social and economic classes of the 'target population' to initiate an active understanding of health."[24]

Since poverty is linked to socioeconomic class, it is important for us to examine the relationship of poverty to dental health care. In New York, a study was done to compare poverty and nonpoverty groups in dental status, needs and practices. Results have suggested that the oral health of the poverty group was poorer than that of the nonpoverty group. The former had more dental problems and these were severe. They also had lower levels of hygiene and less restorative treatment. The poverty group also was more likely to be edentulous and to have higher levels of untreated decay and periodontal diseases. They had more missing teeth, and fewer restored teeth. The study also showed that nearly all differences between the two groups persisted when the data were controlled for age and sex.[25]

Selected dental findings of a rural county in Appalachia showed that 25 percent of the adults had no natural teeth remaining in one or both arches. More women were edentulous than men. Women had more decayed, missing or filled teeth and a lower index for oral hygiene. When compared to the National Health Survey, this sample had much fewer filled teeth, poorer oral hygiene and more evidence of periodontal disease.[26]

The dental profession has made a number of efforts to alleviate the ills of poverty populations. Project Concern, in Appalachia, for example, offered dental services in an equipped van with its home base at Alpine, Tennessee. One dentist and two dental hygientists served the population of most rural areas of eastern Tennessee. The area had had no dental care for generations and the teeth of children and adults were virtually destroyed by decay and infection; emergency treatment was of necessity the project's first priority. After initial emergency measures were taken, patients received a hygiene kit with toothbrushes, toothpaste, soap, washcloth, comb and nail file. Eventually, the patients were taught to accept restorative care and preventive dentistry. On the whole, the project was very successful and arrangments were made with the Tennessee state government for dentists who were licensed in other states to offer their services. In doing so, more care could be offered to a large number of patients.[27]

There is a common assertion that the poor ought to be educated to accept personal appointments and routine comprehensive dental care by a family dentist. A research study[28] had indicated that of 33 missed appointments 14 (42 percent) were mostly due to the clerical errors of receptionists; of the remaining 19 that could be attributed to the patient's "family," eight (or 42 percent) could not be avoided through education as they involved illness or family emergency situations. The remaining 11 cases were attributed to lack of transportation for the disabled and the fear of traveling at night. It was concluded that few appointments were missed because of factors exclusive to ghetto areas; this underscores the need for close attention to administrative procedures in services involving expanded delivery of dental health care to population groups.

Contrary to the public's expectations, the attitudes of patients in low socioeconomic categories can be very positive toward dental health care. A study of the behavioral characteristics of disadvantaged adult patterns in Alabama indicated that dental attitudes were favorable in a majority of the respondents, suggesting that educational and motivational efforts might be fruitful in maintaining good oral health. Many of the patients requested future dental treatment.[29]

A number of studies undertaken in other cultures and societies have shown a relationship between socioeconomic class and dental health care. A survey carried out among 941 members of the Yoruba ethnic group of West Nigeria, for example, was an attempt to find the relationship of periodontal health to socioeconomic status. Russell's Periodontal Index (PI) and the Simplified Oral Hygiene Index (OHI-S) comprising the Debris and Calculus Indices (DI-S and CI-S) were recorded. In addition, an evaluation of the nutritional status of the communities was carried out through studies of the dietary intake and the biochemical estimation of blood hemoglobin, serum proteins and ascorbic acid levels. All of the studies, clinical, dietary and biochemical, showed marked deficiencies of essential nutrients in the low socioeconomic group. The study indicated that while oral hygiene was important, it was vital to consider the patients and their environment in planning prophylactic measures for periodontal lesions. This is particularly essential in malnourished populations.[30]

Research done in Great Britain noted that a lower prevalence of dental caries was found in children living in upper class areas as compared to those living in lower socioeconomic communities.[31]

A population study conducted in Israel attempted to determine dental attitudes and behavior patterns. After the initial study was completed, the findings were compared with those from the United States using an item-by-item analysis. It was found that there were similarities in certain areas: a comparable proportion, for example, reported having a family dentist. The most striking similarity in the two groups, however, was the strong relationship between social class and preventive dental behavior.[32]

In South Australia, the dental health and habits of children from different socioeconomic environments were studied. The results indicated that there was a poor level of dental health in primary and secondary dentitions at all ages and socioeconomic levels. However, children from poor areas had more caries, fewer restorations, more extractions and inferior dental habits.[33]

A study of 300 office and factory workers in Dundee,

Scotland, attempted to assess their level of dental knowledge. In addition, attitudes toward dentists and dentistry were examined. The workers were divided into two categories (manual and nonmanual) with the following results: nonmanual workers were better informed and held more favorable attitudes toward dentistry than manual workers. Consequently, more workers in that category had regular dental treatment checkups and preferred restoration over extraction of their teeth. Alarmingly, 61 percent of the respondents did not know the purpose of fluoridation, the most ill-informed group being the manual workers.[34]

The Underprivileged Patient

About ten years ago, Professor Dummett[35] asserted that the success and efficacy of health care are dependent on the cooperation of the persons who need the care, and that, therefore, it is essential that there be mutual understanding between the consumer and provider about all the factors involved. People are becoming, he continues, very vocal and insistent on being involved with formulating decisions about everything that affects them. He sets out some characteristics of the underprivileged under the following headings:

"Underprivileged" defined: an urban family earning below $3335 per year (in 1969—the figures are approximately doubled for 1980 comparisions). About 41 million Americans were underprivileged by this measure at the time of Dummett's writing.

The poor are different: their reaction to many situations and circumstances are generally different from others.

Hypersensitive attitudes: the matter of dissimilarity between the poor and the non-poor is very important.

Reaction to clinic cleanliness: the aseptic cleanliness of dental clinics and offices is likely to stimulate feelings of personal uncleanliness in the ghetto patient.

Verbal communication: communication between ghetto residents and providers of health care is affected by language differences.

Treatment as last resort: many disadvantaged persons tend to seek medical and dental treatment only as last resort.

Rejection of preventive treatment: explaining preventive treatment to the poor is difficult.

Appointments: the underprivileged are not as unaware of keeping appointments as generally believed; long waits at clinics and at the doctor's office may tend to discourage their keeping appointments.

Fatalism and fear: dental fatalism is common among ghetto residents.

Involvement of the underprivileged in program planning: a primary deterrent to the success of comprehensive health care has been the professional pride and arrogance that effectively insulated the health profession, rendering them distant and self-righteous.[36]

Chapter 4

Race

For decades, the problems of race have concerned many individuals. Yet, the concept of race has not been fully understood by many people. Perhaps the most common mistake is to confuse race with culture, with nationality, with religion, with language or with color. One is likely to hear such statements as "She is a member of a Polish race" or "He belongs to the African race."

In brief, race is not related to language even though the terminology one hears sometimes suggests that it is. For instance, we hear that there is such a thing as an "Aryan" race. Aryans are people who speak Indoeuropean (or "Aryan") languages.

Race has nothing, essentially, to do with geography. There is no "African" race. That is a geographical term.

Race is not to be confused with culture. People sometimes speak of an "Oriental" or an "Occidental" race. Each of these is a cultural designation.

Race is not to be confused with religion. People often speak of the "Jewish" race. This term refers to a religion and a culture. There is no more a "Jewish" race than there is a Protestant, Catholic, Lutheran or Hindu one.

Race has nothing to do with nationality. There is no "Polish" or "German" race. These are nations and irrelevant as far as race is concerned.

Race is not to be known on the basis of skin color alone, although this is a very popular assumption. Some people speak of the "black" race, "brown" race, "yellow" race or "white" race in terms of skin color. The biological components of pigmentation help to identify races, but ascriptions of race involve a greater complexity than skin color itself.

There is no linguistic, geographic, cultural, religious or national group that constitutes a race, *ipso facto*, nor is race to be judged by the color of one's skin.

Race can be viewed as referring to relatively large and relatively permanent subgroupings of humanity whose members share certain selective inherent physical characteristics. Although race has obviously important social and sociological implications, it is a strictly biological category.

On the basis of observable physiological characteristics, the human species is generally divided into three major social groupings: Negroid, Caucasoid and Mongoloid, comprising all but perhaps 1 percent of the earth's human population—leaving small groups especially difficult to categorize. The "unclassifiables" include the Veddas, the Ainus, the bushmen of the Kalahari desert, the Polynesians and Australian aborigines. In many instances, racial belongings are not clearcut, and frequently become even more distorted with the addition of racial myths which may appear to be "logical" on the surface, but in fact originate in and sustain racism.

The real problem, of course, is that race is not so much a biological phenomenon as a social myth. And it is the social myth that causes so much conflict and tension in the United States. A myth may be thought of as a sacred tradition which explains an otherwise unexplainable mystery. It has all the force of reality and serves especially well where other kinds of knowledge are lacking. If people believe something to be real, it will have real consequences for them. Thus, in the case of race we have long used the myth that people were different intellectually, spiritually and socially because they were members of different races. According to this myth some races are believed to be innately superior to others. In this case, then, the myth has served to shape the conscience, to provide a basis for judging right and wrong. Segregating people can't be wrong if they're inferior.

Further, there is a great deal of mythology concerning blood. Many people believe blood is equivalent to heredity and determines the quality of the person, despite the fact that blood of all races involves four blood types, O, A, B, and AB, in differing proportions. It is genes, not blood, which accounts for the transmission of hereditary characteristics. "Blood," however, has become a symbol with real social consequences.[1]

Connected with the symbolism of blood, social visibility or identifiability also operates. The black person, for example, may be thought to be visible for a number of reasons, including "blood" and skin color.[2] Color, however, is determined by the distribution of pigment in the skin. The same chemical pigments are present in all human beings, varying only in their proportion throughout the body. Black Americans have a larger portion of melanin, making their skin "browner" or "blacker"; carotene gives a yellowish tinge to the skin of Mongoloids. The relatively smaller proportion of these chemicals constitute the basis for the beige or "pinkish" skin tones of the "white" Caucasian.

Stereotyping

Although these myths and assertions are false, one must remember that these preconceptions lead to conceptions; what you perceive is largely preconceived. Instead of each individual's being judged on the basis of his or her own merits, people are stereotyped. A stereotype is an oversimplified generalization which emphasizes only selected traits. What is significant in a stereotype of a minority group is that the selected traits tend to be those that emphasize difference from the dominant norm, and make up the whole image of an entire group, thus serving as an excuse for differential treatment. The assumption is that these traits are innate and hereditary and therefore no change in treatment of the stereotyped minority is warranted. Newspapers, magazines and other mass media depend on popular approval for sales; they once were reinforcing agents in the maintenance and continuance of such generalized and popular stereotypes. Stereotyping is the use of a category as invariably relevant. For example, if a successful black man is viewed by a white as not conforming to the stereotype, he might be regarded as an "exceptional" member of his race. Stereotyping of this sort allows unconsciously racist persons to "justify" most unjust behavior. Exclusion of all blacks from a white residential area has in the past and sometimes even today been justified on the grounds that if the "exceptional" family is allowed to enter a neighborhood as a resident, it will soon be followed by black families who are not exceptional but "typical."[3] Stereotyping acts as a vehicle for establishing and maintaining group boundaries; it does not work alone, however. Prejudice and discrimination work with it.

Prejudice and Discrimination

Although prejudice and discrimination are often used interchangeably, they are not synonymous, for a person can be prejudiced against a minority without discriminating against that minority, and can even in some ways discriminate against a minority without being prejudiced. "Discrimination refers to some overt act, some behavior, which selects some attribute (in this case, race) for differential treatment."[4] For example, discrimination takes place when someone is excluded from living in a certain neighborhood, entering a specific occupation or receiving treatment from a particular physician or dentist. Discrimination is commonly "justified" by an assertion on the part of the "unprejudiced" person that he or she has been pressured by peers into conforming to certain standards of behavior; these peers generally use the same excuse. "A person's claim that he is free from prejudice while others have it cannot always be accepted at face value as evidence that an unprejudiced person has been pressured into discriminating."[5] While it is possible to discriminate without being prejudiced, it is not likely.

Prejudice, on the other hand, is not behavior, it is an attitude. "It is the subjective state of the mind of the individual, and need not result in any overt behavior."[6] There are two types of situations in which one may be prejudiced but not discriminating. The first takes place when the prejudiced individual is not afforded an opportunity to discriminate; the second occurs when penalties for discriminating are greater than the desire to discriminate. A store owner, for example, may resent the people he or she is serving in a certain neighborhood but finds business nevertheless to be quite profitable. In most instances, that attitude of prejudice encourages discriminatory behavior.

Prejudice and discrimination affect every institution in American society, including the health care institution. The problems of health care for minority races in the country are real and are, for the most part, common knowledge. They include crowded waiting rooms, inferior facilities, and in some cases unresponsive personnel. Victims of this type of treatment "persistently provide evidence that [the] health care system in the United States is unavailable, unresponsive, unacceptable, and ... to many ghetto residents unimportant."[7]

The process of segregation is another form of urban dynamics in race relations which affects the health care institution. Segregation involves the involuntary residence of persons and groups in a given area on the basis of racial origin, ethnic background or economic level. It is a very complex force involving at times an implicit assumption of inferiority and superiority. Segregated communities almost always evince a poorer average quality of housing, public services, health care and education. A comparison of the white and nonwhite populations in the United States with regard to housing, income, education and employment indicates that despite progress we have not realized the American ideal of equal opportunity for all. Segregation, in the long run, is a cost to the total community. A study comparing the social and economic conditions of whites and nonwhites in 1960 and 1970 reveals that while conditions improved for both groups in the ten-year period, the nonwhites were still significantly below whites in all categories in 1970.[8] Seventeen percent of nonwhites in that year lacked some or all toilet facilities compared to 5 percent of whites; 54 percent of nonwhite males 25 to 29 years old had completed four years of high school compared to 79 percent of white males. Employment figures indicate that 8.2 percent of nonwhites were unemployed compared to 4.5 percent of whites; 21.7 percent of nonwhite male workers held white collar jobs compared to 43.1 percent of white males.

Segregation usually takes three general forms. The first is a voluntary segregation, in which people of the same cultural, ethnic or racial group voluntarily come together in adjacent areas. Ethnic communities in many American cities often called "Little Poland," "Little Italy" or "Little Puerto Rico" are examples of voluntary segregation. A second type of segregation occurs when the clustering is involuntary and the group is arbitrarily forced to live under conditions not of their own choosing. A third form of segregation results when the reason for doing so is economic and impersonal. For example, most white people in urban slums are not kept there by any arbitrary restrictions. The basis for segregation is, to a great extent, economic and impersonal and the members are free to leave the community when they can afford to do so.[9]

A discussion of race must of necessity include an analysis of *ethnicity* since both converge. For example, blacks in the United States are both a racial group and an ethnic group. In sociological terms, an ethnic group is a culturally distinct group of people who are bound together by common ties. The individuals have a sense of common identity, an in-group loyalty, a we-feeling—a feeling of belongingness. In general, ethnic groups live by folkways, mores and customs different from those of the general culture. Members have their own traditions, myths and legends. Their value systems are different from others in the society. Their beliefs are tied to their past and influence their future goals in life.[10]

Ethnicity is most observable in predominantly urban societies where industrialization plays a vital part. The United States has many groups that retain an identifiable ethnic subculture. An ethnic group may or may not be a minority group. At times, the dominant segment of a society may itself be viewed as an ethnic group.[11]

The concept of race is also related to the term *minority*. Marden and Meyer asserted that "to be a member of [a] minority is not only to be a part of a social group vis-à-vis another social group, but to be so within a political unit.... [A]ttitudes of dominant members toward minorities are bound up with a system of values which devalues certain physical and cultural traits.... Minorities are conscious of themselves as groups."[12]

In 1970, racial and ethnic minorities accounted for 12.3 percent of the population of the United States, if persons with hispanic last names are not counted as a minority.[13] Blacks, at 11.1 percent of the population, constituted the vast majority of this minority group, followed by American Indians, and persons of Japanese, Chinese and Filipino heritage.

In the area of dental health care, the number of dental hygiene students from minority groups increased from 325 in

1972-73 to 409 in 1974-75. Each of the above-specified minority groups increased in numbers of dental health students during this period, but the percentage of the total remained constant for some groups because of the increase in students of all groups.[14]

While the number of dental assistant students from most minority groups increased between 1972-73 and 1974-75, there was a slight decrease in the number of American Indian students. The number of Puerto Ricans also decreased in spite of the inclusion of statistics for the University of Puerto Rico for 1974-75.[15]

Although there was a small increase in the number of dental laboratory technology students from minority groups between 1972-73 and 1974-75, the proportion of such students dropped from 21.7 percent to 17.9 percent in the same period.[16]

Race, Ethnicity, and Dental Health Care

Indeed, race and ethnicity are clearly associated with certain kinds of diseases. Since oral health is part of general health and hence affects the total well-being of individuals, it is important that we examine briefly additional aspects of the health care institution in relation to one's racial and ethnic background.

Research has shown that blacks "are less likely than whites to have a usual physician for the children, are more likely to use public clinics for routine and acute illness care and yet are less likely than whites to indicate that children get the best care from the clinics."[17]

Additional studies have indicated that white children and youths are more likely to be considered by their parents to be in very good health and are less likely to be in good or fair health than are their black counterparts. Further, black parents are more frequently worried about the health of their children than are parents of white children.[18]

Significant differences were found between white and black children with regard to the infectious childhood diseases which characterized each group. White children were significantly more likely than black children to have had chicken pox as well as scarlet fever. Black children and youths were more than twice as likely as white children and youths to have had whooping cough. With regard to injuries, broken bones were twice as frequently reported among whites than among black children and youths. Allergies excluding asthmas and hay fever were also reported much more frequently among white than among black children and youths. The proportion of those having frequent colds was significantly less among white than among black children, while the reverse was found with respect to bronchitis.[19]

The study stated further that considering sensory-neurological conditions, black youths more frequently were found to have a history of eye disorders than were white youths. White children and youths, however, had earaches and ringing ears substantially more often than black children and youths. Fewer white than black children and youths were considered by their parents to have speech difficulties. Further, white children and youths were substantially more likely to have had an operation and to have been hospitalized than their black counterparts.[20]

Research on blood-work-ups have indicated that the numbers of parents of children with low hemoglobin values are higher among poverty level families and black families than among more affluent as well as white families. The same pattern holds true for low calorie intake. Also, the average daily intake of calories is lower among children of poor families than among children of familes with incomes above the poverty level, and lower among black children of all socioeconomic levels.[21]

Similar research has shown that over one-half of the black population over 45 years of age have significantly elevated blood pressure levels; only one-third of the white population is in the same position. This discrepancy is most pronounced among females.[22]

An analysis of race and health care further suggests that poor people and minority group members tend to get a higher proportion of their care at hospital out-patient clinics or hospital emergency rooms—*e.g.*, almost 17 percent of the visits for persons aged 17 to 44 in families with less than $5000 income (in the mid 1970's) were at outpatient clinics or emergency rooms, compared with only 9 percent of those in families with incomes over

$15,000. In addition, minority and low-income persons take less advantage of the telephone for procuring medical advice than do nonminority and high-income persons.[23]

With regard to dental health care, studies have indicated that the average number of dental visits is higher for white children than for black children and also higher for families with above poverty-level incomes than for families with below poverty-level incomes. Thus, the children of families with lower incomes have many more untreated decayed teeth and missing teeth and substantially fewer filled teeth than the children of higher income families. The dental health of black children, as compared with that of white children, follows the same pattern. On the whole, many children, especially those in poverty-level families, do not see a dentist as often as is recommended.[24]

A recent study has shown black youths had a substantially greater percentage of periodontal disease than did white youths. The mean PI (Periodontal Index) for all black youths (0.46) was significantly greater than that for all white youths (0.29). When the racial groups were divided into male and female, the trend continued: the index for black boys was 0.45 as compared with 0.31 for white boys, and that for black girls was 0.48 as compared with 0.28 for white girls. The differential also existed among white vs. black youths. Within four of the six age groups, black youths had significantly higher mean PI's than did white youths. Thus the mean PI of black youths was higher than that of white youths regardless of their age or sex.[26]

Another investigation showed that the oral hygiene of white youths was somewhat better than that of black youths. The mean OHI-S (simplified Oral Hygiene Index) for all black youths (1.26) was substantially higher than that for all youths (0.83). In addition, within each of the six age groups, black youths had higher mean indexes than white youths. The differential held when the groups were divided along sexual lines. For example, the mean OHI-S for white boys was 0.92 as compared with 1.30 for black boys. In summary, the mean OHI-S for black youths was significantly higher than that for white youths regardless of age or sex.

In addition to nationwide research, several single state

projects have focused on the relationships among race, ethnicity and dental health care. For example, in a North Carolina project which analyzed the dental health status of a particular group of students (1808 13- to 14-year-old boys) during the years 1966 to 1967, it was found that black students had less dental caries but more oral debris and calculus than whites. Children of both races from the mountainous part of the state had more caries experience than their cohorts from the Piedmont region and the latter had more than those from the Atlantic coast. In all instances, however, children who had used fluoridated water during the first eight years of their lives had less caries experience and better oral hygiene than those students who had no fluoridated water.[27]

A study conducted in Detroit and Columbia, South Carolina, which involved an explorer and mirror examination of 216 white and 429 black Detroit high school students aged 14 to 17 and 349 white and 439 black Columbia children demonstrated that black and white children in both towns had similar caries experience; the mean number of decayed, missing or filled teeth in Columbia was 11.01 and in Detroit 10.42. While caries incidence was higher in white than in black students in Detroit, this was not true in Columbia.[28]

Race, ethnicity and dental care show striking relationships in a number of societies. In Liverpool, for example, 359 children of immigrant parents were examined dentally and 288 families were visited in their homes to complete a dental questionnaire. Black children appeared to show less caries experience and significantly better brushing habits than whites.[29]

In a Canadian study, Eskimos who attended the dental clinic in the Keewatin district of the Northwest Territories were studied for the presence of dental caries. Children examined were from three to nine years old. Dental caries which were very prevalent in the deciduous dentition, were thought to be related to a change of diet and the use of sugar-milk solution in very young children. Decay also was prevalent in the permanent dentition; by 18 years of age approximately a third of the permanent teeth were affected.[30]

A recent study on tooth survival in a variegated group of aged people in Israel has revealed striking results.[31] The study sample consisted of 862 residents of homes for the aged in Israel. The subjects came from a number of ethnic groups: immigrants from various African and Asian-Arab countries such as Yemen, Iraq and Morocco, as well as Europeans from Poland, Rumania and Bulgaria. They all migrated to Israel when already old and lived in institutions; they were more or less insulated from Israeli society and hence it could be assumed that to a large extent they retained the cultures of their countries of emigration. The study attempted to find the percentage of subjects who were dentate according to their specific age, sex, ethnic groups and the average number of surviving teeth. The researchers were interested in getting information on the proportion of those who were toothless vs. those still retaining a number of teeth, the average number of dental units per dentate person and the ability of specific tooth types to survive. They felt that knowledge of these facts would be useful for assessing needs and treatment planning.

It was found that there existed a significantly greater number of dentate individuals among the Afro-Asian group of elderly than among the Europeans. In spite of the fact that economic background as well as access to comprehensive care sources were similar, those of European descent appeared to have higher motivation to make use of available dental services than did the Afro-Asian group—this was seen as a reflection of the "dental attitudes" which existed in each "homeland."

A number of studies cited by the authors supported their finding that elderly patients in advanced societies accepted prosthodontic treatment more readily and, hence, were more prone to retain fewer teeth; for the Afro-Asian group who had less opportunity for access to dental care, a significantly larger number of them usually became edentulous as compared with the European group. The authors concluded that socioeconomic and cultural background influenced motivation to undergo restorative treatment and hence influenced the number of extractions made. In other words, the survival of natural teeth in old age is dependent on access and motivation to undergo dental treatment.

In a study done in West Malaysia which examined the teeth of 15,197 school children aged six to 18, the researchers found variations in the prevalence of dental caries in the permanent teeth of those racial groups involved in the study (Malay, Chinese, and Indian/Pakistani.) Dental caries prevalence was highest among Chinese children (twice as high as among the Malay and Indian/Pakistani children.) Caries prevalence in the Malay and Indian/Pakistani children was comparable. Caries experience in *primary* teeth, however, showed no significant difference for the three ethnic groups.[32] An analysis of the reasons for these differentials in caries experience in permanent teeth revealed that the three most important factors were amount of fluoride intake, oral hygiene habits and dietary patterns and habits. The investigations found that the fluoride level in the water was adequate and could not be implicated as a causal factor; also, oral cleanliness was similar in the groups. The only factor remaining, then, was the diet and dietary habits, which they felt played an important part in causing the variations observed.

Since most of the subjects lived in urban communities, however, the amount of their sweet and sugar consumption appeared to be similar. Thus, the three factors of fluoride intake, oral care habits and dietary habits could not explain the variation in the degrees of caries found in the three ethnic groups. The authors concluded that a genetic difference in the susceptibility of each group to dental caries probably existed. In a similar study cited by these authors, differences in the incidence of caries among the groups were linked to racial differences.

The authors found it more difficult to explain the pattern of caries attack. They concluded that children must be taught to use the dental facilities, which were free but underused, and suggested that increasing the supply of dental manpower could lead to better dental care and ultimately less genetic differences.

Studies done in the United States have shown a strong relationship between racial and ethnic minorities and inadequate dental health care. For example, in an analysis of the oral health status of migrant and seasonal farm workers and their families, it was found that the level of care of the children's teeth was inadequate to prevent future dental problems similar to those experienced by their fathers; the children of seasonal farm workers were shown to receive less treatment than the migrants; the adults had extremely poor dental habits with prohibitive restoration costs. It was suggested that in spite of this high cost, some provisions must be made to prevent these people from suffering pain and infection. In addition, these farm workers must be helped to make the best of existing dental programs, especially preventive ones, and that most significantly, this segment of society must be provided opportunities that would allow their children to escape the cycle of poverty which was their "heritage."[33]

In the United States, several studies attempted to make positive recommendations in order to alleviate the dental ills of racial and ethnic minorities. For example, one such project which investigated the dental status and needs in a poverty population of North Nashville, Tennessee, examined records of 208 patients using the out-patient dental clinic at Meharry Medical College. The racial distribution of the group studied was 93.7 percent nonwhite and 6.3 percent white. The findings, which could be generalized to both ethnic groups, were that even when free services were provided, there was little use of them by these patients; that most of the services rendered them were of the emergency type; however, when additional treatment was recommended, very few cared to return; and that evidence suggested that little emphasis had been placed on dental care in the early formative years of these patients. The study recommended that dental education and motivation should be the prime objectives of dental teams serving in ghetto populations.[34]

A report on the blueprint for the Indian Health Service shows that the goal of such a service is to elevate the oral health of Indian and Alaskan native people, so that no more than six teeth are missing per person at 65 to 70 years of age. This goal, however, necessitates a well-prepared plan. It was pointed out that the quality of program performance is reviewed and evaluated against predetermined standards and criteria. The recipients should be made to feel that it is their program rather than that of the health agency, and that it is carried out in accordance with their wishes and requirements.[35]

Chapter 5

Demography

It is helpful to examine demographic trends in relationship to sociological concepts in order to understand changes in the number of dental auxiliaries in the population, temporary and chronic illnesses suffered by various segments of the population, the concentration of some oral diseases among the impoverished, and the high incidence of other diseases among the wealthy, regardless of race or ethnic origin.[1] In addition, demographic trends point to differences in the quality of dental health care of various social and ethnic sections of the population.

The United States can trace causes and trends of death as far back as the early 1900s. The National Health Survey Act (1956) designated that illness and disability information should be collected on a continuous basis. Consequently the general health of the American people can be accurately evaluated.[2]

Demographers use statistics to demonstrate how certain segments of the population stand at a given time; statistics also deals with the processes that account for population changes and trends over short and long periods of time. People are constantly being born, dying, and changing their place of residence. The basic components of all changes in population, both in time and space, are thus fertility, mortality and migration.

United States Population

The population of the U.S. had grown to nearly 215 million by the middle of the 1970's. This represented an increase of over 1.8 million per year since 1970. Eighty per cent of the increase in population was due to an increase of births over deaths (*i.e.*, the natural increase). Migration is the second major cause of an increased rate of population growth.[3]

The population of the South and West has been growing faster than the population of the rest of the country. In fact, the Northeast and North Central sections of the country have actually declined because of migration.[4]

Women have a lower mortality rate than men. Therefore, the older the population group, the greater the number of women. By 85 years of age women outnumber men by two to one. Between 1960 and 1973 the age of the total population increased, which partially accounts for the drop in the sex ratio of the population from 97 to 95 men per 100 women.[5]

The white population of the United States has a higher average age than "all other" groups. This is due to the lower fertility and mortality rates of the white population.[6]

In the United States life expectancy (for children born at the present time) is likely to increase. All females live an average of eight years longer than their male counterparts, and whites, both men and women, live five to six years longer than others. However, the gap between whites and nonwhites has begun to close.[7]

Population Implications for Health Care

The percentage of degenerative diseases prevalent in the total population has begun to increase with the increase in the age of the population. This has decided ramifications in terms of the emphasis in medical and dental care. New facilities and methods of treatment must be found to handle the increased number of cases of arteriosclerosis, diabetes, nephritis, arthritis and other geriatric diseases.[8]

Although it is not easy to compare the old and the young in terms of acute illness—because restrictions of activity and the like, which are indices of acute illness, may be due simply to age—one can be sure that chronic illnesses are more prevalent among the elderly.[9]

Incidence of chronic conditions such as arthritis, heart

disease and vision and hearing impairments, are 20 percent higher among persons over 65 years of age. Chronic diseases are more often found among elderly who are also poor with the exception of ulcers, which are less common. Forty percent of all people over 65 suffer from arthritis, although it is more often found in women than in men. Women also have a greater incidence of vision loss, back trouble, high blood pressure and diabetes, while men suffer more often from hernias and ulcers, asthma and bronchitis, and hearing loss.[10]

Seventy-four percent of all nursing home residents are over 75 years of age. These individuals are most often female, white and widowed, and 34 percent of all individuals living in nursing homes are residing in the North Central area of the United States. Residents of nursing homes comprise 5 percent of all individuals over age 65.[11]

Nursing home residents under age 65 most frequently suffer from mental disorders (37 percent). Individuals over 65 years of age who reside in nursing homes generally have hardening of the arteries (23 percent), are senile or have suffered a stroke. Circulatory diseases account for 33 percent of all illness among residents of nursing homes.[12]

Three percent of those living in nursing homes are blind but only 1 percent is completely deaf. Speech impairment among nursing home residents is highest for those under 65 years old. One-half of all nursing home residents can read a newspaper without corrective lenses and two-thirds can use the telephone without the help of a hearing aid.[13]

Periodontal disease is the greatest cause of tooth loss in the older segments of the population. This type of dental problem is more often diagnosed among men than among women of similar ages.[14]

Although incidence of tooth loss increases as age increases, the total amount of tooth loss has diminished over time. The amount of periodontal disease rises as people grow older. In general men are more likely to have periodontal problems than women. The most prevalent dental problem of elderly Americans is tooth loss, with poorer individuals sustaining the greatest incidence of missing teeth. Only one-half of all adults between 55 and 74 years of age have any of their own teeth; on the average, 15 teeth are missing of those who still retain their natural teeth.[15]

We can view constructively the various ramifications of health care and population by diagnostically examining fertility, mortality, and migration in relation to space, time and social change in societies. Further, working under the assumption that societies are predominantly dynamic rather than static, one can compare populations at different time periods.

Fertility as a rate or ratio can be viewed in various ways: for example, as a crude birth rate, which refers to the number of live births reported in a calendar year per 1,000 population (actual or estimated at mid-year); gross or net reproductive rates; or the ratio of children (age 0-4) to 1,000 women. It is important to note that fertility is the actual rate at which the population is reproducing and should not be confused with fecundity, by which is meant the potential ability to reproduce.

In the United States the fertility and birth rates are linked to religious and socioeconomic conditions. The fertility rates of whites are lower than those of other races, although the rates for all women in the United States are declining. The highest fertility rates are found in Africa, Asia and Latin America.[16]

There is a great diversity of birth rates among various regions of the United States as well as within each specific region. The highest birth rates are in the mountain states, and there is great diversity of rates in the Pacific states (13.9 to 20.0 births per 1,000 population). New England and the Middle Atlantic states have the lowest birth rates. Nationally, the birth rate declined between the years 1957 and 1973, from 3,724 to 1,896 per 1,000 population for women aged 20 to 24.[17]

Women between the ages of 35 and 39 living in the United States have 3.1 children. The average number of children expected by women who are 18 to 24 years of age is 2.1. The decline in expected family size is not related to educational levels, but is related to age, with younger women expecting to have fewer children in their completed families.[18]

Children born in areas experiencing widespread poverty tend to have a smaller birth weight, regardless of race; 33 percent more white children of low birth weight were born in poverty stricken areas than such children born in other areas.[19]

Many things affect the birth rates of a country or region. The most important factors are cultural. However, economic conditions, health factors, war and deferred marriages also can alter birth rates.[20]

The oldest and in many ways the most reliable measure of the health status of a population is the number of deaths. Death is an either-or proposition and much easier to ascertain than morbidity or illness. Mortality or death rates can also be variously viewed; for example, the crude death rate refers to the number of deaths reported in the calender years per 1,000 population (actual or estimated at mid-year); the infant mortality rate expresses the number of deaths of infants under one year of age per 1,000 live births in a calendar year; the even more limited neonatal mortality rate refers to the number of deaths of infants under one month of age per 1,000 live births. These statistics are the most common measures of health, welfare, and the economic status of a nation. They decrease with increase in economic status of a nation. They also decrease with increases in economic, social, and technological development.

Social factors appear to be most important in reducing infant death rates. The infant mortality rate has been called "one of the most sensitive indices of healthfulness of environment." Koos comments that:

> The plane of living has much to do with infant mortality; a number of studies have shown that, in general, the higher the rent paid by families, the lower is the mortality of infants. Sanitation and a controlled milk supply, together with the education of mothers in methods of infant care, have also much to do with getting infants through the first year of life; all of these are social factors. The death rate in New York City, for example, was lowered sharply after pasteurized milk was made readily available in the slum areas and when mothers were taught proper feeding procedures for their infants.[21]

Within the United States the average lifetime of an individual varies in terms of area of residence. The only state where males' average lifetime is more than 70 is Hawaii. The shortest average lifetime is experienced by residents of the District of Columbia. When the United States is compared with 35 countries having a population of more than one million, it ranks nineteenth for male life expectancy and seventh for female life expectancy.[22]

Educational level and place of residence are related to the death rates of individuals. In general people living in suburbs of metropolitan areas have lower death rates than those living in either rural or metropolitan regions. Interestingly, those who have attended or graduated from high school have a higher death rate than those who have only completed grade school or those who have attended college.[23]

Individuals living in poverty areas generally have a 50 to 100 percent higher death rate than those living in nonpoverty areas. With the exception of New York City this figure does not vary much by ethnic group.[24] It is also interesting to note that the infant mortality rate for white children was 39 percent higher and for nonwhite children 24 percent higher in poverty areas than in other areas.[25]

Migration, the third variable involved in population anaylsis, is the translocation of people. Several types can be distinguished. First, migration may be individual or it may be group; it may also be voluntary or involuntary (forced). Migration can of course be either *international* or *internal* (within a nation). At present most migration in the United States is internal migration on a voluntary basis. Net migration is the result of the difference between *immigration* (migration into a country) and *emigration* (migration out of a country).

If the birth rate exceeds the death rate the population of a nation will normally increase just as if the death rate exceeds the birth rate the population will decrease. If it is true that in most countries, then, under normal circumstances, changes in the population are the result of changes in birth and death rates, still in exceptional circumstances net migration may be so extensive that it appreciably influences the size of the population. The outstanding example of this was the extensive migration of population into the United States during the second half of the nineteenth century.

Social class is related to birth and death rates. The lower socioeconomic classes have more children than the middle or upper classes. The lower class also has a higher death rate than the other groups.[26]

Birth and death rates of a population determine the age of the total population which in turn affects the type of dental care which is needed. Available data indicate that "an estimated 56 million teeth were extracted by dentists in 1969; that there are 25 million people with just 50 percent of their natural dentition, and 30 million people without any of their own teeth; that there are nearly one billion dental carious lessions in the American population."[27]

Recent Dental Care Studies in the United States

Over the past few years several studies have demonstrated the relationship between demography and dental care. One investigation examined the income of dentists by age and location of practice. In 1970 the mean net income of dentists had risen to $29,487, an increase of over 24 percent since 1967. Dentists practicing in communities with a population of 25,000 to 100,000 were the highest paid, as were those practicing in the Far West, and those dentists between the ages of 45 and 49.[28]

Another study has indicated that geographic maldistribution of health care personnel is a major national problem. The State of New York sampled 900 private dental practitioners. Their opinions were sought on several issues including the need for more dentists in their area, willingness to accept new patients and waiting time for appointments. The results showed that 37 percent of the dentists wanted more patients, although dentists outside New York City were less likely to accept new patients than those practicing in the city. It is also interesting to note that patients living outside New York City and its surrounding areas tend to wait longer for an appointment than those living in the metropolitan area. In general the study showed that maldistribution of dental care is a more important consideration than the shortage of dental care.[29]

Given the national maldistribution of dental health care, researchers have devised an easy way to assess the dental health needs of school-age children using a minimum of professional staff and requiring a relatively low budget. Lay technicians, using only tongue blades, note the most serious level of disease in each indivdual. The technicians look for loose or missing teeth, gingivitis, displacements and malpositions of teeth. They also note the number of teeth which need to be restored, as well as those that need to be pulled. The data allow the researchers to estimate the time and cost of dental care needed.[30]

Health Care in Developed and Developing Nations

When populations of societies in economically developing nations are compared with those in more developed countries, they are found to have their own characteristic age structures and patterns of health and disease, which are related to differences in their economic, social, cultural, and natural environments. Many countries are undergoing economic, political, social and demographic changes. These changes are sometimes called "urbanization, industrialization, modernization or development." These factors affect people's lives and their health.[31]

Types of diseases, birth and death rates, infant mortality and migration are not the same in developed nations as they are in developing nations. While the average age of the total population in developed countries is increasing, the age of the total population in developing countries remains rather young, even though these countries suffer high infant and child mortality rates (often, 50 percent of the children born may not survive at age 15). Although infant mortality rates are very easy to control, factors such as malnutrition, gastroenteritis, respiratory infections and pneumonia contribute to the continuing elevation of infant deaths in developing countries.[32]

> From a dental standpoint, malnutrition and starvation are also responsible for higher rates of periodontal disease in developing societies. Deaths from degenerative disease make up a minor proportion of the total because of the few who survive to the aged population. Overall mortality among women is lower than that of men, but higher than that of women relative to men in industrial [developed] societies.[33]

Simple measurement of population growth is insufficient to provide an overview of a country's growth at any time. Some countries have experienced substantial population growth, for example, India, without accompanying institutional changes in the social and economic structure, including the delivery of health care, to support the increased population.

The degree of urbanization, industrialization, and bureaucratization in a society would reflect a community in which there are growing social and organizational complexities. One would expect a more developed nation, rather than a developing nation, to possess the above characteristics to a greater degree. Of course, such characteristics would affect the entire health and delivery of health care to a nation.

If, for example, both a more-developed nation (the United States) and a less-developed one (India) are viewed as of an earlier time, say, 1900, as simpler societies characterized as rural, then by the 1980's the more-developed nation possesses the characteristics of the urban society, but the still-developing nation has little if any change in community organization, persisting as predominantly rural.

In examining the population growth of a nation, it is also insufficient to merely assert that the population has increased; it is also necessary to specify how growth has occurred in rural as well as urban areas. Growth of a population in the urban sector of a nation is often linked to industrialization, with the grouping of industries in certain areas that become job and living centers for large numbers of people. On the other hand, growth in population sometimes occurs with little industialization to support it.

In a developed nation, the relatively large rural but small urban population of 1900 has grown in a pattern of ever smaller rural, ever larger urban, populations. The developing nation begins the same way, with a large rural, and a small urban population, but experiences in later years its growth in numbers almost completely in the rural sector.

A community demographic analysis will help in understanding the health care issues in both predominantly rural and predominantly urban nations. Goals, priorities, and likely outcomes can be more intelligently assessed if such is done. Susser and Watson assert that

> the chance of death fluctuates throughout an individual's life cycle, and the main point of impact of the forces of mortality depends in large part on his or her social and economic background. As the level of production and social organization rises, the main point of impact shifted from the first five years of life to the first year of life, and finally to old age.[34]

Indeed, a community population analysis could, in addition to other variables, strongly help determine the quality and kinds of dental health care delivered in a society. It can also help guide relations between dentists and patients, between dentists and auxiliaries, and between auxiliaries and other health-related professionals. Such analyses are highly significant in understanding and changing the whole spectrum of health services for a society.

Dental Care Studies in Contrasting Societies

Studies in or about cultures and societies outside the United States have also provided some information about the relationships between demographic factors and dental health.

In Japan the dentists-to-population ratio depends on the availability of dental education institutions, the amount of money, influence, and education of local inhabitants, and the modernization of transportation in the vicinity. Therefore the presence of dental disease is not as effective an indication of the number of dentists serving a particular region as is the quality of the life style which the dentist will encounter.[35]

Australian researchers examined the knowledge, attitudes, and practices of pregnant women. They found that there was a relationship between the woman's place of birth and her knowledge of good dental care. The study showed that those born in Great Britain were more informed than those born in Australia. It is also interesting to note that most of the women cited their parents as the chief source of their knowledge rather than dentists or school programs. Although 68 percent visited a private dentist, 71 percent of this group sought the services of their dentist only when they had a specific problem. Fear, money, lack of time, and nonavailability of a dentist were the reasons given for not visiting a dentist regularly.[36]

An investigation done on a limited population in England showed that the individuals studied did not know of the relationship between food debris and dental disease. Oral hygiene practices were also found to be below levels deemed necessary in periodontal practice.[37]

Another investigation, of school children in Finland between the ages of 13 and 16, showed that tooth-brushing habits were generally poor, but girls did better than boys; almost all children had some gingival inflammation; and younger children had less incidence of gingivitis than older children.[38]

As one would expect, the research on health care needs in developing nations has tended to focus on traditional medical concerns with a consequent neglect of problems in the mouth. In the rather infrequent studies of oral disease among people who lack basic health care, the evidence is clear that far-ranging dental care services must somehow be provided. Dietary deficiencies, ignorance of and inattention to oral hygiene, and absence of dental personnel contribute to extensive oral health problems among all age groups. For example, research in a community of Jordan disclosed extensive problems of dental caries, gingivitis, and other oral diseases, inevitably worsening in the absence of dental treatment.[39]

An ambitious investigation of three rural Guatemalan villages involved a diagnostic effort to assess the dental needs of almost 800 people, including 165 children up to 12 years of age.[40] Again, carious lesions were common at all ages; gingivitis, at least of a marginal nature, afflicted many subjects; on the positive side, relatively few children were found to be suffering from malocclusion. Implicit in these findings is the need to explore both the demographic clues to dental care needs and to undertake expanding efforts aimed at prevention and therapy in highly diverse kinds of societies.

Chapter 6

Bureaucracy

The growth and development of formal organizations is a frequently discussed feature of modern industrial societies such as the United States. An important distinction is made between spontaneous and planned activities and these may be equated respectively with play and work. Play activities are, at least in their ideal form, spontaneous, whereas work always requires planning and consequent organization. Anthony Downs defines an organization as "a social system of consciously coordinated activities or forces of two or more persons explicitly created to achieve specific ends."[1]

The more complex an activity becomes the more important it is to plan, and the more inevitable it becomes for a formal organization to be created. The hand craftsman of medieval Europe could produce and sell his products with a minimum of organization because he worked on his own or with a very small number of helpers. The modern city hospital delivering health care to a large segment of a population involves a high degree of planning to bring together elaborate equipment, specialized skills and complex procedures that necessarily accompany scientific advances in medicine and dentistry. All this involves the creation of a complex organization. When certain charcteristics and conditions are present, a specific type of organization develops called a bureaucracy.

Although authors describe the bureaucratic model in a variety of ways, the classic analysis was done by Max Weber. His theory proposed that an ideal bureaucracy has six interdependent characteristics:

division of labor
an administrative hierarchy
a system of standards
impartiality and an impersonal official attitude
employment based on technical qualifications
organizational efficiency.[2]

Weber's concept has been very influential but the defects of bureaucracy have also been pointed out. For example, bureaucracies have a tendency to expand continually. Work expands to fill the time available. Form filling and paperwork are becoming a predominant feature of all industrial societies. However, in spite of all these defects, bureaucracy is the most effective form of administration that has so far been devised.

Technological advances in medicine and dentistry are most apparent in an industriailzed society. In dentistry, new specialists have appeared, each requiring a separate department, so that authority and responsibility can be constructively demonstrated. Thus, departments of endodontics, oral pathology, oral surgery, orthondontics, pedodontics, periodontics, prosthodontics, public health, and many others, have developed over the past years.[3] As a result, the same patient may be served by a number of dentists, both inside or outside a hospital, clinic, or office, as well as by auxiliary personnel.

Bureaucracy is a pyramiding of unit organizations of the social system in any complex society. Bureaucracy contains several subsystems: the authority system, the power system, the status system, the organizational system, the security system, and the role system.

However, bureaucracy does involve a number of related characteristics. These are as follows:

Freedom. The employee is bound by contract to perform various functions during his day's work, but is free to do what he wants after hours.

Hierarchy. The structure of a bureaucracy is in the form of a hierarchy, with each member answerable to a higher authority or authorities.

Competence. There is a high degree of specialization. The members have defined spheres of competence and authority, and the duties and obligations of each group are specifically stated.

Contract. Positions are filled by a contract and both the organization and the individual are bound by its terms.

Qualifications. The various levels are based upon technical competence, often following competitive examinations.

Appointment. The member is ordinarily appointed to his post, with particular reference to his qualifications.

Salary. The salary is fixed for each grade of the hierarchy.

Promotion. Promotion is slow but reasonably sure.

Procedure. The procedure in a bureaucratic setting is highly regularized; communication takes place "through channels" and according to established forms.

Discipline. A bureaucracy is subject to strict discipline. The members are supposed to carry out the work of their office, keep the "secrets" of the organization, and maintain an ingroup feeling against outsiders.[4]

Bureaucracy, therefore, is a "hierarchical form of social organization rationally geared to the achievement of precisely specified objectives by means of a division of labor based on demonstrated competence."[5] This form of organization, Weber writes,

> ... offers above all the optimum possibility for carrying through the principle of specializing administrative functions according to purely objective considerations. Individual performances are allocated to functionaries who have specialized training and who by constant practice learn more and more.[6]

In this connection, Gouldner's analysis of bureaucracy provides a useful extension of Weber's work. As the basis of his research, Gouldner differentiated three patterns of bureaucracy: "mock," "representative," and "punishment-centered."[7] All three types involve division of labor and a hierarchy of positions and rules. What distinguishes one type from another are not these gross bureaucratic features but the relative presence or absence of particular sets of conditions within the broad framework. As Gouldner indicates:

> In *mock* bureaucracy rules are neither enforced by those in superordinate positions or obeyed by those in subordinate positions; joint violation and evasion of rules is buttressed by informal sentiments of participants; and as a consequence there is usually little conflict between the two groups. In *punishment-centered* bureaucracy, however, rules are either enforced by those in superordinate positions or those in subordinate positions and evaded by the other; enforce-

> ment occurs through punishment and is supported by the informal sentiments of relatively great tension and [thus] conflicts are entailed. Finally, in *representative* bureaucracy rules are both enforced by those in superordinate positions and obeyed by those in subordinate positions; there is joint support for the rules, buttressed by informal sentiments, mutual participation, initiation and education of those in both groups; ... a few tensions but little overt conflict occur.[8]

Every organization, therefore, of any significant size is bureaucratized to some degree. Stable patterns of behavior based on structural roles and specialized tasks are apparent. As a general rule it is safe to say that any organization large enough to inhibit face-to-face relationships is a bureaucracy.

In May of 1975 a United States Bureau of Health Manpower was established. The specific goal of this new agency was to give an administrative focus to manpower programs. The Bureau contains several subdivisions, including Associate Health Professions, Medicine, Dentistry, Nursing, Program Development, Program Operations, Program Support, and the Office of Interdisciplinary Programs. Each program includes task analysis, education, training, and continuing education. There are also specialized programs aimed at geographic and speciality distribution of care. One method to implement these programs is the use of student efforts through various institutions.[9]

The health care sector is one of the fastest growing and one of the largest sectors of American institutional life. It should be noted that the U.S. Bureau of the Census gives employment figures on what it calls the "health care industry," but *excludes* people in some health-related occupations (such as pharmacists working in drug stores, nurses working in schools, faculty teaching in medical schools). In 1977, about 560,000 persons were employed in such health-related occupations.

> Between 1970 and 1977, the number of people employed in the health care industry expanded 50 percent, from 4.2 million to 6.3 million. Since the number of employed people in the total economy increased from approximately 76.6 million to 90.5 million or by only 18.3 percent in the same period, the health care industry employment expanded at more than 2.5 times the rate of growth of all employed persons. This rapid growth of a significant employment sector of the economy meant that 1 out of every 7 new jobs ... between 1970 and 1977 ... were in the health industry.[10]

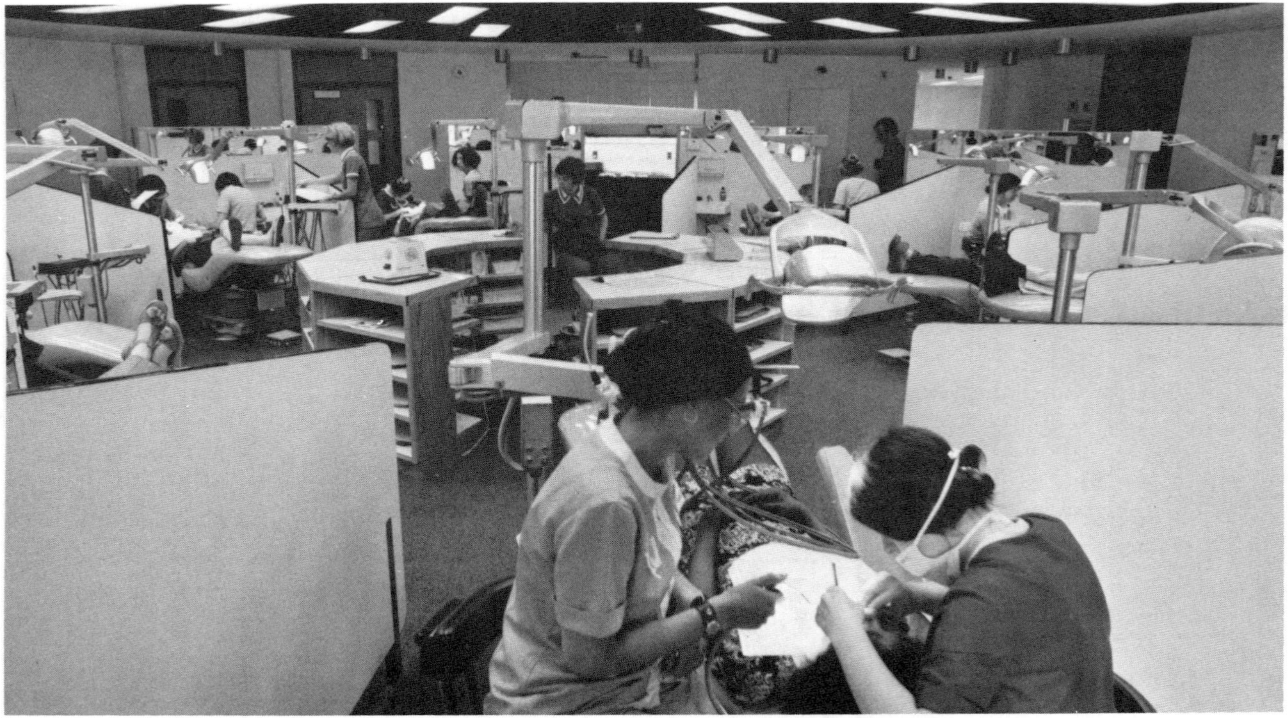

Auxiliaries delivering dental care under the supervision of a dentist (photograph by Ralph R. Lobene)

The numbers of dentists have increased significantly in recent years (from approximately 102,000 in 1970 to an estimated 126,000 in 1980) and will continue to grow (to an estimated 154,500 in 1990), according to Stambler, who says:

> Dental school enrollments and graduates will increase much less rapidly in the future than they did during the past decade and a half. ... First-year enrollments are expected to increase only about 5 percent between 1975 and 1990, as compared with a 59 percent increase over the 1960-75 period. The number of graduates is expected to stabilize by the early 1980s, reaching 5,400 in 1989-90, only a few hundred above the levels of the mid-1970s. By 1990, only 1 new dental school will be added to the 59 that were operating in 1976....
>
> The projected increase in the number of dentists will likely result in a small improvement in the nation's dentist to-population-ratio. The national ratio of 52 active dentists per 100,000 population in 1975 is projected to increase to 60 in 1985 and to 63 in 1990. Between 1960 and 1975 the ratio had scarcely increased, although rising use of auxiliaries such as dental hygienists and dental assistants undoubtedly raised the quantity of dental services....[11]

When many people are added to an organization, a hierarchy of authority emerges. Tensions and conflict arise between the specialist and the person in authority. Both consider their function indispensable and expect their point of view to take precedence, especially in funding. Inherent in the hierarchy is the status system. Dependent on one's position in the line of authority are income, rights, and prestige.

Communications can be a source of problems and irritation within the bureaucratic structure. Communiques such as memoranda can lack clarity, be too long, or be sent too often and therefore lose effectiveness. If methods and forms of communications are inadequate over a long enough period of time, the members of an organization can become irritated, experience role strain and role reversals. Ultimately it is possible that the communication system might break down completely. Communication can be passed along one of three tracts. The formal tract includes official messages, the personal tract is self-explanatory and the subformal tract is a communique that is informal whether or not it is sent through formal channels.[12]

Dental Health Care and Bureaucracy

Since bureaucracy has come to define and to regulate the important functions of all institutions within U.S. society, dental health care has become increasingly transformed into a bureaucratic organization. Indeed, the appearance of bureaucratic administration in almost every sphere of life has not left the dental profession untouched, and this influences all manner of relations among dentists, patients, auxiliaries, and other health-related professionals, permeating dental health services and the community as a whole.

For example, a dental hygienist in a bureaucratic position in a public dental clinic holds her authority not simply by force of her personality, but because her position assigns that specific and limited authority to her. If she vacates her position for any reason, another auxiliary with somewhat similar training and qualifications will move into her spot and the bureau will continue to function. A dental clinic in a large city hospital, for example, has endured in spite of complete turnover in personnel through the years. In order to make this continuity and endurance possible, records must be kept. Mumford and Skipper asserted that "bureaucracy cannot rely on the memories of parts that are replaceable and that have limited authority. The bureaucracy, thus, can offer continuity, order, and a certain predictability."[13] External changes in large bureaucracies also affect dental health care in this society. For example, a dental school must be able to function well with the large bureaucracies that surround it such as insurance companies, corporations that supply dental equipment, and government agencies.

The relationship between dental health education and the institution of government has become increasingly apparent in the last few years. Minority students who were in their first year of dental hygiene training grew from 190 to 227 between 1972 and 1974[14]; the number of black dental assistants increased by 100 for the same two-year period.[15] There was a slight increase of minority students beginning their training as dental laboratory technologists. The only minority groups which showed a proportional increase in dental laboratory technology were those of Asian ancestry.[16] In the six years between 1968 and 1974 the enrollment of women in dental schools was eight times as great as it had been previously. However, women still make up only 6.9 percent of all dental students.[17]

Socially Meaningful Interaction

A medical center in a suburban metropolitan area is another example that depicts the workings of a bureaucracy in relation to health care. Let us briefly describe a Midwestern university medical center to see the interactions in a bureaucratic setting. The center is part of a university complex. With 451 beds and 35 bassinets for the newborn, a hospital has been merged with a large ambulatory care center. The hospital operates a computer system, which is involved in five major on-line applications: Admitting (admissions, discharges, patient transfer, and census), Pharmacy, Clinical Laboratories, X-Ray, and Central Supply. Information is fed through some 30 terminals. Coded carts on an automated delivery system can be dispatched to central locations on every floor for the delivery of food, pharmaceuticals, linens and other materials. Rooms are equipped with regular and closed-circuit broadcasting and a similar setup exists between the operating room and radiology. Although immediate monitoring is done only in intensive care areas, each bedside is equipped for the purpose. Employed within its walls are about 1200 persons daily. A triad of goals forms its purpose: seeing patients through the whole course of their illness and restoring them to their society at a level of optimum functioning, teaching new members of the health team the dynamics of patient care, and researching the illnesses that continue to plague man and investigating newer means for better health.

In order that all members of the health care team understand their purpose, a book of procedures with complete job descriptions was prepared. Three times daily, computer operations send out a patient census, with their profiles as well as categories of patient care to the major functioning areas. These are updated by the nursing team on a daily basis. Although the line of authority is spread on a horizontal plane, it has a vertical dimension as well.

We have asserted previously that before *society-culture-personality* can become functional as an interlocking system, a catalyst or agent is necessary. That catalyst is socially meaningful interaction.

It is important that the dental auxiliary recognizes the implication of socially meaningful interaction, both in terms of quality and quantity, in order to gain an understanding of the health care enterprise. For example, the dental auxiliary should recognize the fact that patients, although presently in seeming isolation, are family members, and their reactions and behavior demonstrate their families' influence on their level of understanding and their attitudes about the meaning and purpose of dental health care.[18] The family, conversely, socializes the patient into a system of dental health care expectations that has been determined by the bureaucratic model. In the socialization process, other agencies, peer groups, and community pressure groups influence the patient's views concerning health and illness.

Health care, an institution within American society, is like other institutions made up of various subsystems or components. Using a dental school as an example, one could identify certain organizational goals such as education, research and dental care services. The implementation of these goals is achieved through a bureaucratic organization that coordinates all tasks. The organizational structure of dental school bureaucracy is composed of a hierarchy of offices and positions.[19]

The board of trustees is the chief policy-making group within the dental school. It is made up partially of community representatives who safeguard the interest of the community within the school. The administrator translates the policies of the board into practice.

Every department and service within the complex has a hierarchy. Within the hierarchy the title and office that one holds confers status upon one, which obviously varies depending upon the job.[20]

The professional person in the clinic organization of the dental institution is exposed to two lines of authority, professional and bureaucratic: both are essential for the functioning of the intricate enterprise. Professional authority rightly demands freedom to act on the basis of professional skill and judgment on behalf of the individual patient in the particular situation, regardless of bureaucracy's rules. Mumford and Skipper noted that "the professional person derives his basic authority from outside the bureaucracy. For example, the nurse and the physician [and indeed the dentist and dental auxiliary] come to work in a hospital [a clinic] with their own professional license to practice."[21]

The organizational bureaucracy has its own network of authority. The medical and dental staff of a health center directs the activities of the personnel (the line). To make the decisions necessary for the center to carry out its primary goal of providing health services, the role of management's authority is reflected in those matters affecting the means of carrying out the doctor's and dentists's instruction.[22]

It is possible to view the bureaucratic connection of each of the components. It may be hypothesized that the interaction between these units will either be associative, tending toward a mutual sharing of responsiblity, power and authority, or dissociative, tending toward tension and conflict situations.

For example, if one considers the variable of power, certain associative or dissociative patterns are apparent. One of the significant patterns in a dental clinic today is the relationship between dentist and auxiliaries. As the recipient of the dentist's orders for his patients, the auxiliary is obligated to carry out those orders in a professionally competent manner, but at the same time, he or she is a hired employee of the institution, and consequently subject to all the rules and regulations of the adminstrative organization. Corwin has indicated that "the tension is severest between professionally-oriented employees and employee-oriented administrations."[23]

Further, the demands of patient care, especially those of an emergency nature, cannot be accomplished within the framework of administrative rules. Thus the auxiliary is in a conflict situation between the expectations of the dentist that his orders be carried out and the expectations of the administrator that administrative procedures will be complied with.

The dysfunctions of bureaucracy were pointed out by men like Veblen, Dewey and Warnotte, who documented concepts of "trained incapacity," "occupational psychosis," and "professional deformation," respectively.

Veblen's "trained incapacity" refers to that condition in which one's abilities function as inadequacies or blind spots, preventing one from adjusting correctly to the changed situation. Thus, skills and training that have been successfully applied in the past may under changed conditions result in inappropriate responses.[24]

Dewey's concept of "Occupational psychosis" is founded upon some observations from the humdrum activities of life in which people develop certain preferences, antipathies, discriminations, and points of interest. By psychosis Dewey means "a pronounced character of the mind." These psychoses originate from demands put upon the individual by the organizing of his occupational role.[25]

However, there are forces at work which tend to lessen the severity of the potential problems resulting from the social structure of a dental organization. Coe asserts that

> One of these is the ideology of service, an historical legacy of the Middle Ages, expressed in modern terms as commitment to a job. A second force is the development of informal groups within the formal organization which permit certain activities to be accomplished regardless of the potential blocks of the social structure.[26]

Insofar as the dentist and auxiliary are concerned, the relationship shifts from time to time and place to place. It varies according to the generation each belongs to, to the size of the community and its dental setting, and to the field of specialization.

Within the past decade, studies have been done to examine several relationships of the auxiliary's role in a bureaucratic structure where specializations have occurred. For example, in order to determine dental students' attitudes toward dental assistants and the possible expansion of assistants' duties, junior and senior dental students from the University of California's Dental School (San Francisco) were queried to form an opinion inventory. The results showed that 83 percent of the students approved of expanding the duties of the assistants (more seniors were in favor of this than juniors). Students having the most clinical experience and those who on previous tests scored highest in autonomy and lack of anxiety seemed to be more likely to exhibit approving attitudes toward the extension of assistants' duties.[27]

Another study depicted the "historical development of the expanded duties of auxiliaries. Subjects include the factors which influence the shortage of dental manpower; controlling influences in delegation of expanded functions; evolution of programs for utilizing dental auxiliaries and the team approach. Topical areas included new responsibilities for the dental auxiliary; programs implementing the expanded-duty auxiliary; expanded functions for the dental hygienists; a review of the education and training for expanded functions; and a review of certification and licensure."[28]

In 1970 Minnesota revised the State Dental Practice Law to allow certain dental services to be performed by trained auxiliaries. Subsequently a study was done to discern the opinion of dentists concerning the expansion of the auxiliary's role in the delivery of health care. In most cases younger dentists were more in favor of the expansion than older dentists; however, respondents of all ages thought that employing an auxiliary would be beneficial. Even though they felt that there would be financial benefits in having the services of an auxiliary, many dentists were still not willing to reduce their fees in order to have their patients share in this saving. Most felt that their patients would accept the service of an auxiliary.[29]

Another study has researched the problems facing hospital dental programs. In the past hospitals have discriminated against dental services and therefore funding of these services was not a major goal. This of course led to problems of obtaining adequate centralized laboratories and the overuse of the facilties that did exist. Another aspect was the difficulty involved in obtaining a sufficient number of staff members in order to provide good services. The study also showed that methods of recruiting interns were often chaotic. Lastly, a major problem facing hospital dental services was the governmental regulations of Medicaid which insist on prior authorization for dental services.[30]

Another study reported the need for greater participation in regional Medicaid programs by dental societies and schools of dentistry. The mission of the regional programs is to "provide a forum and an organizational structure through which health professionals, voluntary and official health organizations and consumers can improve the medical care to the citizens of the nation." The study noted that such emphasis will benefit dentistry if the profession's institutions and organizations will see the needs and grasp the opportunity to foster and support research in the delivery of health care services.[31]

Because of the rapidly growing advances in the field of biomedical knowledge, expertise at the time of one's graduation from professional school can quickly become obsolete. Until recently this aspect of health services had not been adequately researched. Therefore investigators sampled the opinions of dentists nationally to try to determine if obsolescence of knowledge had caused a variation in career patterns, practice, or professional orientation.[32]

The need for hospitals to intensify their programs of continuing dental education has been suggested. Among the topics that could be included in such a program are dental care in relationship to problems of developing an awareness of patients as total members of society, and promoting interaction between dentists and other health professionals.[33]

Studies in other cultures and societies have indicated the relationship between bureaucratic organizations and dental health care. Sweden has a 190-hour core of courses for dental assistants. The primary focus of these courses is general care and they are taken with other auxiliary personnel. The program stresses psychology and sociology. There is also an emphasis on the aging process. An effort is underway to make ordinary radiography part of the duties of dental assistants, therefore radiology is another aspect of the assistant's education. Students seeking oral surgery clinic jobs receive an extra year of training.[34]

New Zealand also has a program for dental school nurses. They have found that very often dental services are more acceptable to children when performed by women. Because of the high status given to women in the program, good students have been attracted to this aspect of a dental career. It has also been noted that a relaxing of rigid supervision by dentists has increased the standard of work performed by the dental nurses. As the program is funded through the government, dental nurses are not permitted to work in the private sector. Children no longer in elementary school but under the age of 17 receive dental care through a private dentist of their choice, and parents always have the option of not using the government funded services.[35]

Chapter 7

The Team Approach to Dental Health Care

A health care team is defined as a group of people with sets of highly developed skills who work together for the common goal of providing coordinated, continuous, comprehensive, correct and compassionate health care for an individual patient.

Implicit in the above definition is the concept of *interaction*. Human interaction occurs whenever human beings respond to the actions of other human beings. Any communication of meaning, by speech, writing, gesture, or other medium, is human interaction. We have noted in the previous chapter that before *society-culture-personality* can become functional as an interlocking system, a catalyst or agent is necessary. That catalyst is socially meaningful interaction. Prerequisites for socially meaningful interaction are social contact and communication.

In the interaction process, each actor takes the other(s) into account, is aware of other(s), and appraises the others(s). However, the process can occur on various levels. For example, interaction can take place between two individuals, between the individual and the group, between the individual and the culture of a society, and between the individual and mass communication.

The quality of interaction will determine to a great degree the effectiveness of health care delivery. Thus, it is important that we recognize the implications of socially meaningful interaction and its subdivisions in terms of the diagnosis, treatment, and prognosis of a patient. Bloom[1] and Evans[2] have elaborated upon the importance of this interaction between the physician and the patient, and their findings can be applied to the dentist, auxiliaries and their patients. The auxiliary should be viewed not as an isolated "helper" of the sick but as a member of a profession that is part of and functionally linked to other cultural subgroups—hospital, clinic, education in general, the American Dental Association, the American Nurses' Association, and economic, social, and familiar groups. Evans has cogently pointed out that health care workers and their patients are products of their culture, regulated by the familiar principle of homeostatis in which no part or function operates independently of all other parts of functions.[3]

Communication, as an element in socially meaningful interaction, is a most relevant concept in health care. Indeed, one of the most essential aspects of care, from the patient's point of view, is communication with health care workers. For example, depending on the way individuals were socialized within their families, they will have certain dental hygiene habits as well as particular attitudes toward dentistry. They may be frightened of dentists and therefore communication between the patient and dentists is vital in order to calm the patient's fears. Patients should be able to communicate with the dentist without fear or hesitation when they do not understand what the dentist is doing or want to ask questions about the condition of their teeth. Dentists in turn should explain to their patients the work they are performing so that the patients can understand the techniques. Through this type of communication, the patient's anxieties and concerns are relieved by the dentist. Hospitalized patients also desire communication with physicians for at least two reasons: first, as a means of obtaining information, and second, as a source of interpersonal contact.[4]

The patient's educational level will affect the ease with which he and the auxiliary can communicate. Research has indicated that the "lower the educational attainment of the patient, the greater the probability that this obstacle [fear of the physician or the dentist] will be a problem and the problem is compounded by limited vocabulary.... Physicians [dentists] may offer explanations to patients, but the message does not get through because the patient is unable to interpret the medical vocabulary."[5]

Interaction is closely related to social processes. Social

processes include accommodation, acculturation, assimilation, competition, and conflict. A knowledge of these processes is necessary to understand the network of relationships in the team approach to dental care. Acculturation, accommodation, and assimilation are types of associative relationships; that is, the individuals are working with each other. At the other extreme, the relationships can be dissociative; that is, the individuals or groups are working against each other. These dissociative relationships are of two kinds, competition and conflict. For example, conflict may arise in a team setting where there are disagreements concerning the proper performances of roles. Role strain may arise because persons lack the necessary skills, talents, or temperament to play a particular role, because role requirements are unclear, or because of a large number of multiple role partners, all with conflicting expectations.

Our perceptions of what other people think of us have an influence on our behavior. It was noted in Chapter 2 that Charles H. Cooley proposed the concept of the "looking-glass self" to describe this process which is linked to interaction in a team setting. Thus, we not only have an idea of what other people think of us but we also have feelings about ourselves contingent on that perception. These feelings about what we think other people think of us cause us either to continue our behavior reinforced or to modify it.

The Team Approach and Dental Health Manpower

Health manpower is and has been for more than ten years a growth industry. The size of the overall workforce is now more than 50 percent larger than it was in 1960. By 1990 it will be nearly 8 million workers—almost three times the 1960 figure.

Up to five million persons were employed in health-related occupations in the 1970's. One-half of these were in nursing or related services. There was one physician for every 562 persons in the United States in 1973. The number of individuals to be treated by each physician ranges rather widely among industrialized nations; several nations, including the U.S.S.R., Israel, Italy, and Hungary, had larger numbers of physicians in relation to population than the United States. Other nations, including Canada, Sweden, France and Great Britain had more persons per physician than the United States. Some countries with longer life expectancies than the United States had relatively fewer physicians.[6]

The milllions of health care workers are often categorized into two major manpower groups—health professionals and allied health workers. Although the first group of health professionals that generally are recognized include physicians and dentists, the largest number of health workers actually are nurses. There were nearly 860,000 registered nurses employed in the United States in 1973, as compared with 340,000 physicians and 107,000 dentists. On the other hand, there were only about 19,000 optometrists and only slightly more than 7,000 podiatrists.[7]

The other major groups of health workers are in the allied health fields. Allied health workers provide essential supporting and technical services to health professionals and health care institutions. In 1973, nearly three million persons were employed in the allied health fields in such occupations as clinical laboratory technologist, physical therapist, medical record technician, occupational therapist, dental hygienist, dental assistant, dietetic and nutritional services, radiologic technology, etc. The allied health field has expanded even more rapidly than the health professions in recent years even though the latter is more well-known. In 1973, for example, the number of dental hygienists and dental assistants were 21,000 and 116,000 respectively.[8]

The proportion of health professionals who are of one racial or ethnic background or another varies widely by profession. For example, fewer than 3 percent of physicians and dentists in the United States are black. However, over 20 percent of dietitians and practical nurses and 40 percent of lay midwives are black. On the other hand, fewer than 2 percent of all dental hygienists and about 4 percent of all dental assistants are black.[9]

Since auxiliaries will be working with dentists from the standpoint of the team approach to dental care, it is important to examine the number of dentists in relation to population and specialities. There were 100,000 active nonfederally employed dentists in the United States in 1973. The supply of dentists in relation to population only slightly improved between 1960 and 1973, from one dentist for every 2,138 persons to one dentist for every 2,088 persons. The greatest increase in the proportion of dentists in relation to population occurred in the West, South, Central and Mountain states.[10]

Dental Group Practice

The concept of dental group practice plays a vital role in the team approach to dental care. From a historical perspective, the first dental clinic or closed panel of dentists was formed in New York City in 1790. The next 100 years saw many changes in the practice of dentistry. The dental schools established their own clinics or dispensaries for the care of the indigent. It was not until the early part of the 20th century, however, that the many types of current group practices of participating dentists began to emerge. Since World War II an ever-increasing trend toward group practice can be seen in dentistry.[11]

There are many definitions of group practice as applied to modern dentistry. The Bureau of Health Manpower Education has adopted the following definition: "a *group dental practice* is defined as a practice formally organized to provide dental care through the services of three or more dentists using office space, equipment, and/or personnel jointly."[12]

Dental groups meeting this definition are further classified on the basis of one of the following types of fields of practice:

> *Single specialty groups* are those providing services in only one field of practice or specialty (other than general practice) or including less than one full-time equivalent of another specialty.
>
> *General practice groups* are those composed exclusively of general practitioners or of general practitioners with the addition of less than one full-time equivalent of another specialty.
>
> *Multispecialty groups* are those composed of practitioners in two or more fields of practice with at least one full-time equivalent in a field other than general practice.[13]

According to the 1970 Public Health Service survey of dental group practices in the United States, there were 3,148 dentists identified as practicing in 715 dental groups. More than three-quarters of the 3,148 dentists were employed full time in group practice.[14]

Nearly two-thirds of the dentists practicing in dental groups were general practitioners; a bit over 10 percent were oral surgeons and nearly 8.5 percent were orthodontists.[15]

There were 7,358 "auxiliary personnel" employed in the 715 dental group practices in 1970. The Public Health Service survey defined auxiliary personnel as all nondental personnel employed in a dental group practice. On the average, slightly more than two auxiliary personnel are employed for each dentist in group practice. Dental assistants account for almost half the auxiliary personnel employed. Secretaries and receptionists account for another 23 percent.[16]

Additional studies have been done on dental group practice. One dealt with a comparison of solo and group practices; some of the conclusions made were these (the percentages are rounded):

> solo dentists are less likely to employ hygienists: about 62 percent of them had no hygienists as compared with 42 percent for group practitioners; the latter group employed "some" hygienists more often than the former group (58 vs. 38 percent).
>
> dentists in group practice also employ more staff; their use of auxiliary and support staff increases with the size (*i.e.*, the number of dentists) of practice.
>
> dentists in group practice report higher income than those in solo practice.
>
> on the "index of attentiveness to professional activities outside practice," dentists in group practice are found to be proportionately more active than those in solo practice.[17]

Another study analyzed the benefits of group practice over solo practice for patients as well as for dentists and auxiliary personnel. The quality of work done for patients in group practice is greater at minimal cost to both patients and practitioners. It was the researcher's point of view that group practice is better for society as a whole, for it can render quality service to all segments of the society regardless of their socioeconomic backgrounds.[18]

A similar study divided group practice into the "mixed" and the "pure" types. A "pure" group of either all general practitioners, or all specialists. The "mixed" type is thought to provide better comprehensive dental care, for it attracts dentists of varied talents who can provide different types of service.

Advantages of group practice were noted by the author of this "mixed" vs. "pure" study; in general they are the following. Modern managerial techniques and machines facilitate dentists' routine work, leaving them free to devote more time to serving the patients. Since dentists in group practice can combine their credit ratings and are able to share costs, they are able to purchase the most modern dental equipment, the use of which brings greater benefits to the patients at reasonable costs. Auxiliaries are more efficiently employed in more responsible duties in a group practice environment; this helps to relieve dentists from routine work so that they can devote more time to patients. Peer review becomes possible in the very organization of group practice, which makes quality control a basic aspect of the duties performed by group members.[19]

The Comprehensive Care Concept

The best of modern knowledge and skill delivered to and applied to individual patients constitutes "comprehensive care." It is a planned and supervised flow of services and resources leading to an ongoing program of health promotion, maintenance, and restoration. Within the concept of comprehensive care, the idea of prevention must be available to complete the spectrum of service by the many interdependent health disciples and specialists. Implied in the teaching of health is the promotion of health and its maintenance. Both the well person and the patient as a consumer assume some responsibility to absorb and to use the information communicated to them.

The holistic approach to health is implied in comprehensive care, which calls for the exercise of skill and judgment in the integration of various services required to meet the needs of individual patients. Holism demands that attention be given to emotional and to social, familial and physical factors, and continual monitoring, without overwhelming the patient, in the hospital, clinic, or home until he or she is safely through convalescence and rehabilitation. The availability of health care for all people requires

> an information system which can signal the health care needs of the country; an educational system which can supply adequate numbers of well trained persons of the right type; a coherent set of common perspectives which would stimulate the health professionals to work together; and an organizational network within which these workers can form collaborative relationships.[20]

One study suggests that new concepts for group practice of the future are necessary so that dentistry may fulfill its goal of providing treatment for everyone. Some of the suggestions that were given include comprehensive care, construction of clinics for all types of prediagnostic testing, employment of technicans and all types of paradentists, and the expansion of duties for auxiliaries so that repetitive work can be eliminated for dentists. The study forecasts that comprehensive care in dental clinic systems will be the trend of the future; in such a system both dentists and auxiliaries will be playing an increasing role.[21]

The Team in Action

The team concept requires a number of people to work together as a team in order to achieve a common goal. This implies interdependence, a full utilization of skills, and the exercise of coordination for internal efficiency and external representation. As a team develops, there tends to be a shift of emphasis from the depersonalized professional and technical roles to the personal contribution of these important shared skills. Matters discussed become less "medical" decisions or "dental" or "nursing" decisions. Instead, other team members are expected to assist with their own informed perspectives and personal support. By exercising their special skills, the team members can produce right courses of treatment. The dynamics of the health team are focused on considering the full range of patient needs, involving a comprehensive approach, both patient-centered and family-centered.

Over the past decade several studies were done to explore the attitudes and values of auxiliaries as team members in the delivery of dental care. For example, one study explored a dental hygienist's changing self-concept when she becomes a practicing member of the dental hygiene profession. The importance of unified political power and of the influence of the practicing hygienist are examined. The American Dental Hygienists' Association's policies and communications are considered important to the realization of dental hygiene's ideals as they relate to the public and the profession.[22]

Another research study examined the social attitudes of hygiene students from the viewpoint of professional concerns and services to the disadvantaged. A sample of 108 dental hygiene students was investigated on the basis of the sociopsychological aspects of social class backgrounds and selected attitudes; the data were gathered through questionnaires and attitude inventories. The findings provided information about the students' high school extracurricular activities, their primary reasons for entering the profession, important factors in achieving career satisfaction in the profession, and their opinions about the most important problems facing the dental profession today. The latter question identified the major difficulties as the manpower shortage and the delivery of dental care to the indigent, the aged and the disadvantaged. Attitudes toward location for practice and job satisfaction were related to the concern for the poor.

The project further analyzed various attitudes of these students, especially their willingness to serve in areas where poverty was widespread. Those students who were concerned with the indigent, the aged, and the disadvantaged were more likely to seek employment in economically depressed areas. Approximately 5 percent of the respondents were unwilling to leave their present position regardless of the type of offer.[23]

Several studies have examined the functions of the auxiliary as a member of the dental health care team. One such study reported that if the desired adequate system of delivery of oral health services for the United States is to be attained, a system other than the present one must be devised. Currently, the system perpetuates the pattern of concern over the productivity of the dentist but not that of any other dental health care worker. Two reasons are given for the reluctance of dentists to change the current practice pattern: professional competition (from other dentists who may well be trained for example, in cavity preparation and tooth extraction, which are most demanded by clients), and fear of loss of economic security.

The findings of the above study concluded that dentists should be prepared to delegate duties to auxiliaries, who were deemed capable of becoming as proficient as dentists in such functions as restoring teeth with plastic materials and routine teeth examination. The hygienists could be trained to prepare cavities, perform plastic restorations, and extract deciduous and permanent teeth. Such functions would not lessen the professional authority of the dentists; rather, they would free them to perform those oral health duties requiring a higher level of skill than auxiliaries have.[24]

Another study examined the professional aspirations and job satisfaction of dental assistants who are given expanded duties. This study investigated the effects of the expanded duty movements on those auxiliaries experiencing it and showed that trained dental assistants can be a valuable asset in reducing the manpower shortage in the existing American dental health care delivery system. This alleviation can be brought about by encouraging the professionalization of assistants through their involvement in accredited dental assistant programs and continuing education programs designed to expand their skills. A high percentage of expanded-duty auxiliaries seemed to indicate a generally high level of occupational satisfaction. Support of professional aspirations for dental assistants can lead to positive outcomes in the effectiveness of the team approach in the delivery of dental care as well as the easier attraction of more qualified individuals to the dental assisting field.[25]

Another study focused on the perceptions of dentists and dental students in Minnesota where dental practice acts allow expanded duties for dental hygienists. The older dentists were less likely than dental students and younger dentists to favor the delegation of new duties to auxiliaries.[26]

An experimental program in expanded functions for dental assistants was carried out in 1971. In the third phase of the study many of the tasks usually done by the dentist were delegated to trained dental assistants and evaluation of their work was then carried out. The experimental aspect of the project extended over a three-year period. The productivity and efficiency of the dentist working with four assistants was compared with the dentist working with only two or three assistants. The dental assistants in this program were given extensive and intensive training and were assigned to do certain procedures: pumice prophylaxis, adult and pedodontic radiographs, and carving of complex amalgam restorations. Although the time required by the dental assistant to carry out these tasks was far greater than that required by a dentist, as their period of training was lengthened, the time element decreased. In phase I, the time required by a dentist to accomplish a complex amalgam carving was five minutes; for assistants in phase II the time was 12 minutes and in phase III, seven minutes. When all procedures were taken into account, the time required by the assistants to complete procedures in phase II was found to be about 70 percent more than the time required by the dentist in phase I. In phase III, the time required by assistants to complete procedures was lessened but they still required about 40 percent more time than the dentist. The quality of the work done during this phase by the dental assistants was evaluated and more than four-fifths of the procedures during phase III met the required quality standards. The quality standards set for the project were extremely high and all the dental services provided met the basic requirements for good dental care. The quality of dental care was examined by independent evaluators.

Patients treated by dental assistants tended to be satisfied with the care provided by the assistants. The team productivity was evaluated and it was found that a dentist working with four assistants performing expanded functions increased productivity by 110 to 130 percent. When the dental team was reduced to one dentist and three assistants with expanded functions, the productivity increased over the baseline performance from 62 to 84 percent. The data of this project supported the concept of using dental auxiliaries to perform a wide range of services traditionally done by the dentist.[27]

One group of authors noted their prevous involvement with an alternative method to group practice. The method was called the "satellite office" concept, which allowed cooperation among dentists who still retain their separate offices and practices. Their attempt to utilize the satellite office requires full-time management and dentists with organizational skills, which they were unable to provide. The authors dropped the concept as premature in favor of group practice; they note the importance of well-trained auxiliary personnel in the success of group practice.[28]

Another study documented the role of the dental hygienist in preventive periodontics.[29] A group of 42 freshman and 38 senior dental hygiene students were questioned to analyze the effectiveness of preventive periodontal education in the dental hygiene curriculum. One year after graduation the students were again evaluated for possible changes in attitudes and preventive practice. It was shown that the dental hygiene education program is effective in teaching preventive periodontal care to dental hygienists.

However, the hygienists do not or cannot fully use this knowledge and skill, because of the attitudes prevalent in dental practices in which they are located. Although there is a great need for dental hygienists in preventive dentistry, a depressing picture emerged. Indications are that 86 percent will resign from full-time employment five years after graduation; 42 percent will have remained in for only one year. Basic changes were indicated in dental education: the causes of attrition or abandonment should be determined, retired hygienists should be encouraged to continue practice, consideration might be given to recruiting and accepting men for education as hygienists, and the dentist's concept of the hygienist's potential role ought to be appreciated and clarified.

Research has been done emphasizing the importance of training auxiliary health workers for effective performance in dental services. Duties for health aides include communicating with consumers of health services, identifying personal health care, promoting good health habits and performing general administrative tasks.

Professionals who supervise dental hygienists or assistants require special preparation to enable them to understand the philosophy behind the use of auxiliary personnel and the new health career movement, and to understand their role as a health team member. Specific behavioral patterns, knowledge, skills and attitudes required of the trainees should be identified so that they may perform the desired tasks effectively. Educational experiences needed for teaching the desired knowledge, skills and attitudes should be determined and carefully planned so that they will relate to productive outcomes. Educational materials for training as well as teaching methods should be selected carefully and integrated into the lessons. Training programs should be planned and implemented in the order that is most meaningful to the trainees. The effectiveness of training can be determined by measuring the student's achievement at the end of the course using behavioral objectives determined at the beginning of the program as criteria for evaluation.[30]

Another study stated that full utilization of currently available dental auxiliaries should be encouraged, and the hygienist should start to occupy three new roles: a new dental health educator, who could provide motivation for treatment; a dental auxiliary educator; and an associate to the dentist who could perform both technical and judgmental tasks.[31]

The role of the dental auxiliary was further analyzed in those areas where dental care needs of the United States are surpassing the potential of the nation's current system to serve them. More dental auxiliaries are needed to relieve the dentists of time consuming tasks. The findings centered around two major options. The roles of existing auxiliaries—dental hygienists, dental assistants, and laboratory technicians—can be expanded to include tasks now performed by the dentist, or a new auxiliary position can be created for this purpose. The study traced the historical background of the role of the dental auxiliary, illustrating some of the pros and cons of each alternative as stated by the American Dental Association, dental hygienists and other dental health care workers.[32]

One study of the expanded functions of dental auxiliaries as members of a team noted that the auxiliary has been severely limited in duties. With a modest amount of additional freedom, auxiliaries can assist the dentist to treat more patients to a greater extent or to treat more patients in a given amount of time. This can be done without compromising the quality of the service given, the ethics of the profession or the welfare of the patient. A listing of permitted duties must be determined. There will have to be a method by which official supervision of expanded functions can be conducted and additional educational facilities to train the auxiliary personnel developed.[33]

The Team Approach in Other Cultures

One author states that group practice is far more common in Yugoslavia than is solo practice. He notes that among certain advantages to group practice are reduced costs of operation and cooperative work. From the psychological standpoint, the author notes, cooperative efforts may become strained between group members because both the dentists and the assistants have different temperaments and characters; income distribution may aggravate the situation if practitioners in group practice decide to equalize their incomes, meaning that individual ability, hours worked, tasks performed, etc., must be taken into account. A grouping of dentists, assistants, hygienists, and auxiliaries may bring about stress as is typical of large groups, including disturbances involving interpersonal relationships, differences in approach to practice, inequality in patient loads, differences in "honoraria" collected, etc. The authors suggest that psychological testings be given to all dentists who decide to form a group in order to determine whether each is temperamentally suited to cooperative efforts. Rooms should be made available to permit needed relaxation for dentists and assistants working long hours.[34]

Another study noted the increasing economic pressures (costs of equipment, building, surgery rental, staff salaries, laboratory charges, etc.) on all types of private dental practice in New Zealand. The private dental practitioner must, therefore, pass the costs to patients in the form of increased fees which can result in a gap between the need and demand for dental care among the population. A solution to this problem involves an increased efficiency in private practice with practitioners delegating simple duties to auxiliaries. The authors of this study felt, however, that leaders in the dental profession in New Zealand only pay lip service to such delegation. A trend that is emerging within the United Kingdom and the United States is group practice, which is almost totally absent in New Zealand. There are many benefits to be gained from group practice, one of which is a more efficient use of auxiliaries.

The above authors felt that conditions in New Zealand may not favor the largescale group practice employed in Los Angeles (which provides dental care to employees of the Los Angeles Hotel-Restaurant Employees Union Welfare Fund), but smaller scale group practice principles can be adopted in New Zealand's larger cities. Such practice will increase the efficiency of dental care because it will provide a structure into which operating auxiliaries can be utilized. The New Zealand Dental Association should be, it was felt, more openminded about the more effective use of hygienists and other auxiliaries and about improving dental practice in the country by adopting group practice.[35]

In Canada, another author sees the objective of the dental profession as providing more services to the public at lower costs and higher quality and feels that the team concept of dental practice calls for the use of auxiliaries to their fullest capacity so that more services can be provided at reasonable fees. He states that:

> the time come for the extensive delegation of our responsibilities in dental care. In fact, the most desirable evolutionary trend for Canadian dentistry is toward rapid establishment of community-oriented group practices which fully utilize dental auxiliaries in the provision of preventive dentistry.[36]

The dentist should delegate duties in his office to auxiliaries who have specialized in various tasks so that comprehensive care can be provided to the people.

Chapter 8

The Community and Dental Health Care

A community can be defined as "that combination of social units and systems which perform the major social functions" in one locality.[1] It is the place or setting where institutions function. The behavior of a community subsystem is greatly dependent upon the quality of interaction among its institutions; the institutions, in turn, are affected by their community setting. Thus, there is a reciprocal relationship between the health care institution, on the one hand, and the community, on the other.

A community has two basic elements: "It occupies a particular territory and the members share a common sentiment. There are three main components of this community sentiment. The *we-feeling*, by which the members of a community tend to identify their interests with the interests of the group, is one; another is the *role-feeling*, through which community members have a sense of place within the group and feel that they have a role to play. A third is the *dependency-feeling*: the members come to depend upon the community for physical and psychological satisfactions. It is a refuge from solitude and from the fear that accompanies the isolation of the individual characteristic of much modern life and activities.

The most important characteristic of a community appears to be *locality*. We have noted in the first chapter that two community types, the *Gemeinschaft*, or rural community, and the *Gesellschaft*, or urban community, are of particular relevance.

In a rural community, social order is "based upon consensus of wills, rests on harmony and is developed and enabled by folkways, mores and religion."[2] The individual is closely tied to other member of the community by family and cooperative relationships as well as by folkways, mores and religion common to the rural group. Family is the basis of life in this type of community; the village and town can, in a sense, be considered as large families.

The folk community is characterized by isolation, homogeneity, lack of communication, conservatism, and traditionalism; it, like all communities, is faced with the problem of providing medical and dental care to their population. The shortage of dentists and auxiliaries in this type of community reflects the small and scattered population, the isolation from colleagues, the smaller incomes, and so on.

The rural dweller's relative physical isolation, desire to avoid intrusion by outsiders, and lack of adequate medical and dental facilities lead to serious health care problems. For example, "during 1969-70, there were an average of 1.5 visits per person [throughout the United States] per year. Persons living outside the central cities in metropolitan areas had the most visits for dental care, 1.8 per person; the rate decreased to 1.1 visits for farm residents."[3]

The urban community, on the other hand, is the result of the industrial-technological revolution. In an urban community, or *Gesellschaft*, social order is "based upon a union of rational wills" and "rests on convention and agreement, is safe-guarded by political legislation, and finds its ideological justification in public opinion."[4] The *Gesellschaft* member is less strongly tied to his family because outside interests tend to separate him from family members. Cooperative relationships are contractual in nature, tending to conceal hostile or antagonistic interests, for there are few common understandings, customs, or beliefs to create a common bond. Whereas inherited property is one of the most important differentiating characteristics in a *Gemeinschaft*, earned wealth is the most important differentiating characteristic in a *Gesellschaft*.

The urban community may be examined in four basic divisions, namely, development, structure, ecological processes, and urban life and personality.

Development

The need for food, water, and transportation are essential factors for the location of an urban community. The city is an ancient type of social grouping, having originated over 5,000 years ago in, it is held, the Middle East, but it is only in the last century that certain areas of the world have become predominantly *urban* in character.

According to Burgess, the central shopping and business district of the city has the highest land value. This is the area where the department stores, museums, theaters, city halls and hotels are found. Almost inevitably, Burgess concluded, the economic, cultural, and political life of the city is concentrated in the center.[5]

Over the years, the growth of cities brought about certain revolutionary social changes. These include the division of labor rooted in specialized skills, a social organization based upon one's status or position in the community, trade and commerce, government as an institution, and an efficient means of communication.

Structure

Clear patterns of behavior are apparent in the relationship of one individual to another. It is all such ordered patterns of social actions and interactions that form a *social structure* in the social system of a community.

Although each community has a different social structure from that of others, the structures of all communities have common features and this allows analysis of communities as such. The structure of a community can be viewed in many ways. Three of the most sociologically useful involve patterns of urban design, urban sprawl, and racial imbalance.

Patterns of Urban Design—These include several ecological theories, and the most fundamental seems to be Burgess's well-known theory of concentric zones. Burgess asserted that cities grow through a process of expansion in which the population flows outward from the center. The central business district is surrounded by zones of generally better-class residences.

The first zone is the central business district. Surrounding this area is the zone of transition where small businesses and factories can be found. Here one finds rooming houses and low-priced hotels. In the days of high immigration, this was an area of settlement for many foreign-born workers. It is in this zone that ghettos are most likely to be found with a high concentration of crime, delinquency, disease, poverty and broken homes. This is also likely to be "skid row."

The area within the third zone contains the working people's homes. Dwellings are somewhat better than those in the zone of transition. The second-generation immigrants inhabit this zone so that they may remain in close proximity to the industries that employ them. There is hardly any clearcut separation between zones II and III. The zone of transition gradually blends into the third, with the housing becoming more improved as one moves away from the center of zone II.

As workers gain more security, they move farther out where single-family dwellings and exclusive apartments are found in residential areas. This is zone IV where one finds grocery stores, drug stores, cleaning shops and beauty parlors. The area contains fewer children, and there is a higher per-capita income.

Finally, beyond the city limits is the commuter zone, the suburban areas or satellite cities. People who can afford the cost of commuting to and from work live here. It is typically the residential area of prosperous businesspersons and professionals.

Urban Sprawl—The expansion of the city limits into suburban areas has meant that the surburb, which is economically and culturally dependent upon the city, has grown faster than any other type of community.

Racial Imbalance—The migration of whites to the suburbs and an increase of the black population in the city produces a racial imbalance in both areas.

E. Franklin Frazier documented the fact that Chicago's black families lived in a long, narrow, rectangular belt beginning just south of the downtown area. He asserted that the poorer black newcomers to the city were concentrated in areas close to the center of the city. Assimilation into urban life and the attainment of relative wealth and prestige were associated with outward movement.[6]

Ecological Processes

Human ecology is the study of how people and institutions are located in space. Human ecology emphasizes the place of the institutions in the community and their relationship to each other.

Closely related to ecology is the concept of *social process*, because ecology emerges primarily from processes of competition and mobility. Social processes, by definition, are special forms of interaction that occur with regularity and uniformity.

In the analysis of the community, human ecology plays a very essential role. The ecologist is directly concerned with problems of transportation, sanitation, pure air, and the distribution of people and institutions.

Urban Life and Personality

The culture of an urban setting is much the same irrespective of geographical location. All cities have social problems such as crime, delinquency, drug addiction, poverty, and poor health care facilities in some areas. All have subcommunities which retain some rural customs and traditions.

However, there are degrees of difference between urban and rural communities and no community can conform totally to either of these extreme types. Some of the major characteristics of these two "ideal" or "pure" types of communities are as follows:

Rural	*Urban*
The family is consanguine	The family is conjugal
Division of labor is based on age and sex	Division of labor is based on specialized skills
Social control is through intimate groups	Social control is through the state

Communication is personal	Communication is impersonal
Social organization based on	Social organization based on
Primary associations	Secondary associations
Personal relations	Secondary groups
Conformity	Impersonality
	Tolerance
Population is homogeneous	Population is heterogeneous
Status is ascribed	Status is ascribed *and* achieved
Setting is a village or town	Setting is a city or metropolis

Another feature of the community is the distinction between *ruralites* and *urbanites*. The former have their roots in the community and tend to take a greater interest in the institutions and affairs of the community. Urbanites, on the other hand, are geographically and socially mobile and are concerned with various issues outside the community in which they reside.

The concepts described in the preceding pages demonstrate the dynamic interaction between the community on the one hand, and institutions on the other. We shall examine more closely the relationship between the community and the health care institution—specifically dental care—as it affects the lives of individuals who inhabit the various communities.

Poverty and Health in the Community

The persistence of poverty among one-fifth of the American population, with increasing numbers of people with low incomes and inadequate savings, has placed greater demands on the health professions to provide high quality and compassionate health care for all citizens.[7] Indeed, such a demand represents an essential part of the United States effort to remedy the plight of the poor in various segments of the population.

Research on the community has helped to increase social and political awareness of health and poverty. These studies have identified different standards of medical and dental care designed to fit two main segments of the population: private practice, which essentially serves the middle class, and public clinics, mainly serving the poor within the welfare system.

The rural sector of a community seems to be affected most with a lack of quality and availability of medical and dental care. Although there have been vast economic and population changes over the past decade, over 50 million American people still live in rural areas. With an average of 380,000 individuals returning to rural America each year, the problem of rebuilding lost health services becomes more essential. It has been asserted that "today, health care is a critical problem in rural areas [where] low population density, high proportions of elderly, poor or uneducated citizens, poor transportation ... combine to make access to health services difficult in many areas and impossible in others."[8]

A recent study by the National Center for Health Statistics has indicated that irrespective of location, racial minorities usually experience poorer health than do whites. The report also showed that minorities in poverty areas have a higher infant mortality rate than whites (about 33 deaths per 1,000 compared with 24), a greater percentage of illegitimate births, greater lack of parental care and higher death rates from tuberculosis and violent causes. The same figures are higher for minorities than for whites in nonpoverty areas. In brief, people who lived in urban poverty areas were subject to death rates 50 to 100 percent higher than other people.[9]

From the standpoint of family health expenditure, research has demonstrated that income spent on personal health services is highest for low income families. "For families with incomes under $2,000, 12.6 percent of family income was consumed by health care in 1970, and only 3.5 percent for families with income of $7,500 and over."[10]

In analyzing the health care of a community it is important to note that in 1974 two-thirds of all expenditures for personal health were handled by third-party payments. Medicare and Medicaid paid about 38 percent of the health care bill, while 26 percent was covered by private health insurance. Medicaid expenditure in 1974 amounted to $11.3 billion dollars with New York, California and Illinois accounting for 41 percent of the total, while "8 other states received 30 percent and 43 remaining states only 28.3 percent of total U.S. medical assistance payments."[11]

Since dental care is tied into the general health care of a community, it is important to look into factors surrounding the uninsured population and the various allocations of health expenditures.

In 1970, 23 percent of the United States population were not covered by hospital insurance. About 44 percent of the uninsured population were 17 years of age or under. Few of the uninsured were over 65 years old. However, 50 percent of the uninsured were below the near-poverty income level while only 14 percent of the insured population were below the near-poverty level. In brief, the uninsured could be described in 1970 as relatively young, low income, poorly educated, and urban.[12]

In 1974, the United States spent approximately $104 billion for health care. This amount represents four times the amount spent in 1960, and approximately eight times the amount spent in 1950. Hospital care had the greatest increase in health expenditures. In 1940 only 25 percent of all health expenditures were for hospital care compared with 40 percent in 1974. Over the years, the proportion of all health care dollars spent on physicians, dentists, drugs and other services had decreased because of the large increases in hospital and home care.[13]

Selected Research Studies

In 1973, the American Dental Association reiterated the basic goals and ideals of the dental profession in helping to organize state, federal, and local dental care programs. In terms of the community, the report dealt with optimal means of organizing maintaining, financing, and defining eligibility of recipients of local community dental health care programs. The report was quite general and dealt directly with a few specific organizational problems.[14]

Along similar lines of inquiry, another study focused upon implementing effective local community health care programs. The following points were emphasized: the need to accept the fact that access to health care is no longer the privilege of a few, the need for full cooperation between consumer (patient) and provider (dental professional) about all the factors involved, and the effective utilization of the "return of the native," *i.e.*, attracting the "young, bright ghetto and rural residents" who train for medical and dental careers and then move back to their community. The study, in general, adhered to a policy of "stop, look and listen": stopping the rapid development of extensive and sophisticated reconstruction techniques (and emphasizing preventive dentistry), looking at the commitments of the health community to improve the health status of the American people (meaning there is a serious need to get more dentists into the community—therefore the time period for completing training programs should be drastically reduced), and listening to what the disadvantaged are saying as well as to what the affluent are thinking.[15]

In another statement, the same study discusses the concept of "extramural programs in community dentistry." It applauds the "trends of extramuralism," *i.e.,* allowing dental students "the opportunity to acquire an appreciation for the wholeness of the individual as a dental care concept, together with an understanding of the community of which the individual is a part."[16] The study also discusses the "MEED" (Multiphasic Experiences in Extramural Dentistry) program established at the University of Southern California, and how it is the most appropriate for the "extramural" approach.[17]

In a study dealing with preventive dentistry, it was argued that with the increasing interest in the practice of preventive dentistry, dental professionals must view themselves as part of the "whole fabric of a community educational-economic-legislative-social system." Professional individualism is no longer important and dental hygienists are now becoming actively involved in working with many different community groups in a variety of human relations activities related to their dental skills. Therefore, there is a move toward—and a great need for—in-service training programs for dental professionals to emphasize human relations and organizational development skills.[18]

Again, emphasis is laid upon the need to develop a "new sense of priorities" on the behalf of the dental practitioner. It is suggested that along with this new sense of priorities new skills will have to develop. Since the major new priority is community-oriented rather than individual-oriented health and dental care, dentists must become adept at total community assessment, and must develop new skills in leadership and management. Interestingly enough, one "management skill" the study carefully delineates is the need for adapting the organization of the practice to the collection of professional fees from third party payees (*i.e.*, government agencies).[19]

From the standpoint of community dentistry and periodontology, a study pointed to the necessity of a change in the priorities and values of the American dental profession and emphasized cooperation among members of the health team, with the government, with all dental schools, with auxiliary personnel, and with the community as the key to successful and effective delivery of dental health care.[20]

A description of a special elective course at Howard University noted the effectiveness in training dental hygienists (very effective) and the delivery of preventive and restorative care (moderately effective). The study suggests that training in expanded functions for the dental hygienist (*e.g.*, preparing a simple cavity and placing restorative material) would benefit the community in terms of total preventive care because the hygienist in a preventive capacity is uniquely situated to handle these needs.[21]

Research focusing upon community involvement suggested that since the dental hygienists' prime functions are community service and education they have a special responsibility to investigate the facilities available to all sectors of the population. The study goes on to demonstrate what the organization might be for a volunteer program to provide adequate care for the exceptional child (those children with visual or auditory impairments, the brain-damaged, the emotionally or mentally retarded, the mongoloid child, those with neuromuscular diseases, and with bleeding or cardiac disorders).[22]

In England, the establishment of a dental care project at the London Hospital Medical College dental school was based on the assumption that the provision of dental care should be considered in a logical sequence. The steps involved were (1) the definition of the community for which dental care is to be provided, (2) the determination of its dental needs and demands by epidemiological methods, (3) the design of the dental team or teams best fitted to meet those demands and needs within the limitations imposed by available resources, (4) the establishment of such a team or teams within the community, (5) the determination over a period of years of the community's changing needs and demands, (6) the assessment of the effectiveness of the team or teams in achieving the objectives for which it or they have been designed, (7) the redesigning of the team as appropriate.[23]

Given the seven points above, it is of interest to note the findings of a report of a week's visit to a community by two senior dental students at the University of London.[24] The visit was part of their undergraduate training in understanding how a community lives and works; it was also to help prospective dentists grasp their role in the community.

Fourth-year students at the London Hospital competed by submitting a three-minute radio script on dental health; one student was chosen and another nominated. The two students stayed in a private house in the community of Taunton, making them feel like part of the community, rather than like mere visitors. The students were left free to pursue whatever interested them, ask questions, make notes, and take photographs. They visited homes, agencies, and dental centers, and observed various general dental practices. Some basic health statistics were provided them beforehand, together with copies of a comprehensive official guide.

The visit was essentially a public relations one and was a success; the hosts were evaluated as to their attitudes toward the visitors in terms of the students' manners, dress and bearing. These factors were rated by the hosts highly and perceived as a credit to the dental profession. For the students, they mostly enjoyed themselves, learned a great deal about how a community functions, and how individual dentists fit into the overall pattern. They were asked to prepare a report which was passed on to other students.

Because the students' visit brought various groups in Taunton together during regular evening meetings arranged principally for their visitors, rapport was achieved among these groups, which included general practitioners, hospital consultants and public dental officers, even after the students had departed.

Another study done in England measured restorative dental care in communities.[25] The Restoration Index (RI) indicates the level of restorative care within a community; it is a ratio of filled teeth to filled plus decayed teeth. It is believed that the RI can be used to measure the level of restorative care in any community at any age.

A survey of dental health in England and Wales in 1968 showed that the RI for the north of England (in a population of 401 dentate persons) was similar to the 72 percent national average; in London and the Southeast (in a population of 593 dentate persons) the RI was 68 percent for the irregular attenders. In general, the higher the social class the higher the restorative care; this was shown to be true in all districts studied.

Similar community studies and determination of respective RIs were done in two northern communities: York (with low fluoridation) and West Hartlepool, a fluoridated community. The RI for York was 94 percent, higher than that for England and Wales (72 percent) and London and the Southeast (80 percent); the RI for Hartlepool was 70 percent. The dentist-to-population ratio in West Hartlepool was 1:8700 as against 1:4600 in England and Wales in general. The communities in England and Wales were all nonfluoride or low fluoride; thus Hartlepool was able to achieve an RI equal to the national percentage with fewer dentists; part of this is due to the fluoridation of the water in West Hartlepool.

The research compares the findings with studies in the United States showing dentist-to-population ratios of 1:2000 with an RI of 82 percent for whites and 41 percent for nonwhites. Given a standard demand rate for dental treatment, universal fluoridation could mean that the present level of restorative care in England and Wales could be achieved by fewer dentists per unit of population.

Fluoridation and the Community

In 1973, a review covering a 30-year span of systemic and topical fluorides for the prevention of dental caries was carried out. The study noted that about 150 million people in 30 countries were then drinking well fluoridated water: the United States had 92 million of this figure. The study also reported that the Republic of Ireland has adopted legislation for natural fluoridation; Japan, Poland, the U.S.S.R. and Yugoslavia all show good progress in the same direction, while Hong Kong and Singapore are 100 percent fluoridated.

The study asserted the fluoridation constitutes an ideal public health program conferring benefits to all, regardless of social status or dentist availability. Any program aimed at prevention of caries must adopt fluoridation as basic to all other techniques. An important point raised in this direction is that mere installing of fluoridation equipment in public water supply is not enough; continued checks must be made to ensure that the proper amount of fluoride is discharged into the water distribution system. The study cites various findings as to how fluoride can be made available to children who live in fluoride deficient areas.

It revealed that some studies have been based on the hypothesis that the prevention of dental caries can be enhanced by part-time (*e.g.*, on school days only) and belated (beginning at age 5 or 6) exposure to higher than optimal levels of fluoride. These studies demonstrated that school fluoridation confers greater benefits (less caries) to earlier erupting teeth (incisors and first molars). Enough studies have been done confirming the safety and the efficacy of school fluoridation that it can be justifiably accepted as a public health measure in areas lacking in central water supply.

One method of administering fluoride is daily consumption of fluoride-containing tablets, but various studies show that dental caries can be best prevented when fluoride tablets are given to children during a regular school day. Fluorides were first administered in salt in Switzerland in 1946 and some research findings confirmed the effectiveness of this salt-based fluoride. Milk was also used as a vehicle of fluoride administration and some positive caries prevention resulted. Topical application of solutions containing fluorides helped to inhibit caries if properly applied. The 1973 review study recommended there be more investigations into various methods of self-applying fluorides by children as well as adults.[26]

In England, research findings on the benefits of fluoride in drinking water concluded that life-long studies are needed to uphold or refute the statement that fluoridation is helpful only to children. The study made a reexamination of previous studies based on two communities in the north of England, one with optimal fluoridation (West Hartlepool), the other, York, with very little fluoride in the drinking water. The sample of people consisted of those who had lived continuously in the towns. An analysis of the sites of attack in the different teeth (maxillary and mandibular) were made and classified by age groups.

The findings showed that several other population factors must be considered to assess the life-time effects of fluoride in drinking water, one of which is the life span of teeth. Also, loss of teeth in a fluoride community is less than in a low fluoride or nonfluoride community. The study finally documented the point that fluorides in drinking water have substantial life-long benefits.[27]

Innovative Community Dental Care

In 1974, a study focused upon the responsibility of the hospital to multiphasic community dental care. The findings suggested that the modern hospital must become an increasingly important place in which the dentist functions. The dental education largely provided in the United States has resulted in making dentists strangers in the hospital because traditionally and through practical necessity, the major concern of dentistry in the hospital has been oral surgery. Hence, oral surgeons are better able to function in the hospital than other dentists, who usually feel inadequate and uncomfortable in the hospital setting.

The role of the general dentist should be to understand the diagnostic laboratory services available in the hospital and how these services can be used to provide total dental care to the hospital patient. Dental students should view the hospital as an integral part of the educational experience so that they may be better prepared to take on their role in the hospital setting. In the light of modern concepts of comprehensive dental care related to the whole patient, it is no longer acceptable to provide dental care or to teach clinical dentistry in isolation from any overall health consideration.[28]

The same study also considered the community hospital as rapidly becoming the health center of American communities. Thus dental care should not be limited to provision of toothache-oriented emergency service or just oral surgical service, but a complete department of dentistry must be opened in the hospital for comprehensive dental care. Many hospitals, such as Mount Zion Hospital and the Medical Center in San Francisco, have long supported broad-based hospital dental programs.

The study noted that a large number of people could not obtain comprehensive dental care because of the difficulty of transportation, inadequacy of private dental offices, physical incapacity, etc. A hospital with the proper dental facilities and trained paradental personnel can make a big difference in overcoming these problems. Setting up dental programs in a hospital does not require a great expenditure of money. The study calls attention to the "health maintenance organizations," which have been growing for some years; there are group practices which are hospital-based, and they reach out with satellite clinics to neighborhoods or nearby communities.[29]

Another study looked at the University of Connecticut's School of Dental Medicine and their new program of preparing students to work in group practice situations. For the first time in over 125 years of dental education, a dental school was integrated with a medical school. Dr. Lewis Fox stated:

> I think dentistry, in the truest sense, is a specialty of medicine.... I looked to the year 2000 and saw certain changes in dentistry on the horizon. I believe dentists will become more related to hospitals, and a lot of new arrangements will ensue. It is to this end that we aimed the curriculum at Connecticut.[30]

One study called attention to government policy, which has, since 1974, created and invested area health authorities with the responsibility for administration of health care under the National Health Services. The study concluded that area dental officers will play a key role in the operation of dental service; they will direct salaried dental staffs, maintain liaisons with the dental teaching hospital, and provide needed dental service to both the area and the local health authorities.

Area dental officers will need data from their districts necessary for the development of plans. Thus, the aim of the study is to describe a method for obtaining such data from a health district. The data, obtained by both dental examination and interview, give a profile of dental health status, use of dental services, and attitudes toward dental health among the total population of the borough. Such data can help to determine, by classification of subjects, whether any required treatment can be carried out by ancillary personnel or whether a dental surgeon is needed. Also, interview questions can assess utilization patterns, knowledge of disease processes, motivations for seeking care, whether group practitioners are preferred to clinic or hospital facilities, etc.[31]

The British Dental Association is increasingly bringing to the attention of the dental profession the need to extend its traditional responsibilities so that not only their patients but also the community at large will be able to benefit from their services. Community-based dentistry typifies the dental profession in England; eight out of every ten dentists work in general practices within the communities. The dental profession, therefore, needs a more effective organization to carry on its duties in these communities. Since the needs of the communities vary from one area of the country to another, local planning rather than national goals should be formulated in order to achieve effectiveness of health care delivery at the local community level. An initial step toward this goal is the forming of an area dental advisory committee. The committee would have an obligation to advise the area health authority on the development of dental services in the area. The committee would need information on the dental needs, demands, and resources of its area, expert advice, and practical strategies. The area dental officer must be able to collect and present practical information useful in the planning of health services, knowledge of both cost-effectiveness and the efficiency of modern methods of dental treatment and preventive techniques being foremost among the officer's qualifications. The area dental officer must also be familiar with the whole range of social and health services in order that dentistry can be seen to play its rightful role in community health.[32]

Chapter 9

The Elderly and Dental Care

Old age is a phenomenon to be found in every society, be it *Gemeinschaft* or *Gesellschaft* in orientation. In the past century there has been an excessively rapid growth of the aged population. In 1970, Americans 65 and older numbered 20.1 million, or one in eleven—more than 17 times the number in 1870. During the same period, the total population increased by only a factor of five. The end result was a faster rate of growth for the aged population and a major increase in the percentage of the aged in the total population. In 1900 there were only 3.1 million people age 65 and older in the United States but by 1940 the number had tripled. In 1975, those over 65 totaled 22.3 million or one in ten. The number is increased by approximately 300,000 to 400,000 per year so that by the year 2000 it is expected there will be about 29 million persons ages 65 or older.[1] There also has been a rising ratio of women to men. One of every eight females is 65 or older, compared with one of every 11 males. The number of older people in the mid-1970's was approximately 13 or 14 million women and nearly 10 million men.

Marital status is one of the primary factors determining living arrangements and family status. Among elderly men, 79 percent are married, 14 percent widowed, 5 percent single and 2 percent divorced. For elderly women, the figures are 52 percent widowed, 39 percent married, 6 percent single and 3 percent divorced. Seven out of ten individuals live in families; only 4 percent live in institutions. Eight out of ten older men live in families, two-thirds of which include a wife. Six out of ten women live in families. One-third of older women and one-sixth of the men live alone or with persons other than relatives. Over four million of the elderly live with relatives other than their spouse.[2]

Almost two-thirds of the country's elderly live in cities or suburbs, the rest in small towns or rural areas. The biggest segment lives in the South, followed by the Midwest, Northeast and West. In metropolitan areas, the aged are generally concentrated in the central cities. Ernest W. Burgess long ago noted this trend in his concentric zone theory of urban ecology.[3] In 1969, approximately 60 percent of the population 65 and over lived in metropolitan areas, and more than half of those lived within the central city itself. An even larger proportion of nonwhite elderly live in central city areas.[4] In towns of 1000 to 2500 populations, over 12 percent of the population are elderly; many farmers move to nearby towns after retirement.[5]

About 20 percent of the aged are foreign born; about the same percentage are second-generation Americans. Thus, almost two-fifths of the elderly population are foreign born or children of foreign born parents, with some likelihood of divergent cultural backgrounds or actual conflict of cultures. Some of the elderly speak English with difficulty or not at all. Fewer than 8 percent of the total elderly population are nonwhite, which is less than the expected proportion since nonwhites comprise about 12 percent of the total population; put another way, almost 10 percent of the white population but only a bit over 6 percent of the nonwhite population are 65 or older.[6] This indicates the much higher mortality of the nonwhites.

As for schooling, the elderly are not so well educated as the majority of the population. The median number of years of schooling for the elderly is about 8.5 years, slightly above an elementary school education. The median for the total population 25 years old and over is almost 12 years. One of five elderly persons is functionally illiterate, with fewer than five years of formal education. For the entire population, one of 14 is functionally illiterate.[7]

In the mid-1970's families headed by an individual 65 or older had a median income of $7,298 a year, compared with $12,836 for all families and $13,645 for families headed by a person in the 55 to 64 age bracket. One of every six older people is classified as poor. Almost 70 percent of the elderly poor are women. Among blacks, 36 percent of the elderly are poor, compared with the 14 percent for elderly whites.[8]

The total governmental expenditure for older people amounts to well over 100 billion dollars annually—more than one-quarter of the federal budget. Included in the above amount are Social Security and other retirement benefits, supplemental-income payments, food stamps, Medicare and Medicaid.[9]

There are basic social and human needs which affect the elderly. Besides the sheerly physical needs, Fromm identifies five basic human needs that persist in society throughout the life cycle: a sense of identity, a feeling of relatedness or belonging, an assurance of "rootedness" (place to which one can feel attached), a confidence in transcendence of our time-limited existence, and a frame of reference to organize life (a religious belief or philosophy of life which provides a system of explanation for the observations and experiences that otherwise seem unexplainable).[10]

Self-realization, the need for recognition, affection, social approval, independence, and self-reliance are other often-used descriptors for basic needs. The aged also share a need for emotional security, to love and be loved, to retain their participatory roles in society, to be productive if at all possible, to receive recognition for their accomplishments and efforts, to have a voice and a choice in the way their lives are lived, and to maintain a feeling of dignity and self-respect.[11]

Old age can be a time of role surrender; it can also be a time of role change. The loss of work role and the child-rearing role, combined with declining physical vigor and economic resources, make up the framework of the disengagement process that is regarded with anxiety and apprehension by the aging.[12] Unless a positive reordering of previous roles is achieved or alternative new roles acquired, the trauma of "role exit" can be devastating. It has been documented that "the negative impact of role losses and the feelings of helplessness and uselessness engendered may account in part for the high incidence of depression among the elderly and the staggeringly high suicide rate for elderly white males."[13]

Activity vs. Disengagement Theory

In the gerontological literature, there are two general points of view with regard to optimum patterns of aging. As noted by Maddox, "with few exceptions, research in the United States has consistently supported the hypothesis that, among the elderly, maintenance of contact with the social environment is a condition of maintaining a sense of life satisfaction."[14]

This first view, one that might be called the "activity theory," implies that, except for the inevitable changes in biology and in health, older people are the same as middle-aged people, with essentially the same psychological and social needs. In other words, "successful aging" can take place only if the older person resists the narrowing of his or her social world, maintaining the activities of middle age as long as possible, and then finding substitutes for those eliminated.

In the disengagement theory, as originally described by Cumming and Henry,[15] decreased social interaction is a mental process, one in which both society and the aging person withdraw. In this model, successful aging would take place when the aging person accepted or even desired decreased social interaction. The disengagement theory implies that a new equilibrium between the individual self and society must be established. The needs of the individual combine with the new needs of society on a basic functional level. A detachment or disengagement of this older individual from past patterns of social interaction is necessary in an ongoing society.

From the above brief summaries of the two theories, the point in contention is clear: activity must be maintained or increased to compensate for the narrowing social world of the elderly or activity must decrease along with the narrowing social world.

The Impact of Age on Physical Health

The older person retains most of the same physical and psychological needs of a younger person, the difference being that certain of these needs diminish and others heighten with advancing age. It must be remembered that not all aged are sick. Shanas noted that in a sample of 1,400 persons, only one in five felt that his health was poor; four in five described their health as "fair" or "good." Yet among these same persons, it was reported that "seventeen out of twenty had had an illness or health complaint during the four weeks prior to the interview."[16] Thus, the majority of the older population of the United States view themselves as being in good health despite the high prevalence of chronic conditions and impairments and high utilization of health care services. Only a small number consider their health to be poor. Minorities, residents of the South and nonmetropolitan areas, and persons with low incomes are more likely to view themselves as in poor health than their counterparts.[17]

The elderly are not a homogeneous group. They differ in their social-psychological outlook, financial condition, temperament, ability to handle difficulties, self-assurance, and physical vigor. The aging process varies from person to person and within an individual from one organ system to another. Furthermore, the aged comprise three rather distinct groups. People from 65 through 74 are usually in better financial condition, health, and housing than their elders. They tend to be slightly better educated, more capable of dealing with social and personal problems. Those 75 through 89 years of age tend to be less well off, not covered or inadequately covered by Social Security, less well physically and emotionally, less capable of making plans without assistance. The oldest segment, those aged 90 and over, tend to have less opportunity and ability to communicate their needs to others and to be less well physically. They are often the most socially isolated because of the prior deaths of family and friends.[18]

Overall, disease and disability rates rise with age. Mortality rates rise too. Among persons aged 75 to 84, for example, the death rate in 1973 was 79 per 1,000 persons. Fifty years earlier, it had been 119 per 1,000 persons. Even though the death rates for diseases of the heart has been declining since 1950, this is still the leading cause of death, as it has been since the statistics have been available. In 1973, diseases of the heart accounted for 46 percent of the deaths in this age group. Malignant neoplasms and cerebrovascular diseases each accounted for about 15 percent of the deaths. These three causes accounted for 63 percent of all deaths reported for these people.[19]

Dramatic declines have been noted for influenza and pneumonia as causes of death. Rates for deaths due to accidents and to arteriosclerosis have also declined over the past 50 years while rates for congestive lung disease deaths have increased.[20]

One of the major indicators of the long-term impact of chronic illness is the limitation of mobility. Approximately 3.5 million persons, or 18 percent of the aged noninstitutionalized population, have some degree of mobility limitation, with about one-third of such persons confined to the house because of their illnesses, another third needing help of a social aide or other person to get around, and the remainder having at least some difficulty getting around alone. This is in addition to about 960,000 aged persons living in nursing homes, most of whom have some degree of mobility limitation. The major causes of mobility limitation among the aged are arthritis and rheumatism, impairment of the lower extremities, heart conditions and stroke.[21]

From the perspective of dental morbidity, it is important to restate the fact that periodontal disease becomes increasingly prevalent among men as they advance with age. During the later years of life, it is the leading cause of tooth loss. Only about half of the adults 55 to 74 years old have any of their natural teeth left. Among those who still retain some teeth, the average number of missing teeth is about fifteen.[22]

Certain bodily changes, not always apparent, occur with aging. A decrease in energy and resistance capacity because of a decrease in actual cell number is characteristic of the aging process. An older individual can often maintain physical balance under normal conditions, but he or she has inadequate reserves to meet the increased needs imposed by the stress of disease.[23] Aging lungs, for instance, show decreased elasticity, as does the chest wall, due to infiltration and deposition of collagen. Thus, the aged person's rate of air exchange is reduced to almost half the capacity enjoyed at age 30. Aging kidneys show a decreased function, a lowered ability to remove wastes from the blood, because the number of kidney cells has similarly decreased as compared to the number in the person's prime. Moreover, the blood flow to the kidneys is reduced about 50 percent because of lower output and higher arterial resistance arising from cholesterol deposits. The aging heart functions less effectively and is more frequently subject to arrhythmias and irregularities in electrical conduction to rhythm.[24] Decreased functioning of the endocrine glands reduces the effectiveness and interaction of hormones and so the coordination of the metabolic process. This phenomenon is exaggerated in times of stress. There is decreased utilization of glucose, even of large doses. Decreased adrenal activity—and so decreased adrenocorticotropic hormone—hampers one's ability to adapt to stress situations. The basal metabolic rate is decreased to approximately 84 percent, thus accounting in part for lower body weight. And with the drop in the total number of functioning cells, the remaining cells must function at maximum capacity.

The cells of the nervous system begin to die early in life. Unlike other cells, nerve cells are not regenerated. As one ages, the time required for nerve impulses to travel across synapses is increased; consequently, specific responses are delayed. The main detriment to the nervous system is to the brain itself, not to the peripheral nervous system. There is decreased brain weight, representing cell loss, ranging up to 44 percent of previous size. Loss of function is especially great in the area of recent memory. Blood flow to the brain is decreased by 20 percent per unit of remaining brain cells.[25] Reduction of acuity in vision, hearing, taste, smell, touch and balance is common with aging, as is a reduced ability to handle complex activities and unfamiliar tasks.[26]

Other bodily changes with aging include skeletal changes, a slower rate of healing, and slower reponse to infection. Decreased elasticity of blood vessels can result in circulatory changes; decreased circulation to the lower extremities is common. A progressive diminution of the ability to withstand stress (accidents, disease, and severe psychological events among them) is another physiological manifestation of aging.[27] Diseases of the heart, cancer, and vascular lesions affecting the central nervous system (*i.e.*, strokes) account for about 75 percent of the deaths of individuals over 44. Accidents among the elderly are also frequently the cause of, or prelude to, death.[28] Illnesses and chronic conditions such as arthritis, hypertension, arteriosclerosis, nephritis, emphysema, bronchitis, and acute respiratory diseases like pneumonia become ever more common with added years.[29] Unattended periodontal disease results in loss of teeth among many of the elderly, especially with neglect of this presumably "natural" happening.

The elderly are often faced with radical, disruptive changes; almost as often, these occur suddenly and simultaneously. Older people encounter the multiple needs to accept failing strength, sensory and motor disabilities and other handicaps along with loss of many friends and relatives. Is it at all surprising the "elderly cope less easily and adapt less well" to stress? Without substantial and constant support, they can easily feel isolated, overwhelmed and helpless.[30]

The Impact of Age on Mental Health

In addition to all these physical consequences, the biological changes of aging affect the elderly individual's self-image. Changes in physical appearance (*e.g.*, wrinkled skin, thinning, graying hair, loss of teeth), slowing reaction time, early onset of fatigue (real or "escapist"), decreased keenness of the senses, debilitating disease and loss of memory are difficult for an individual to accept. In this youth-oriented culture in which physical vigor, beauty, and swiftness of movement are valued, such changes can lead to depression and rejection of the individual by self and others in society.[31] Assistance on many levels is often needed if adaptation and maintenance of a healthy self-concept are to be achieved. Changes in interpersonal relationships often occur rapidly, even simultaneously. Perceived uselessness of self to family and society, felt rejection by and loss of some contemporaries, difficulty in holding old and making new social contacts, loneliness and fear—these compound the elderly person's difficulties, increase depression and add to the sense of helplessness.

The elderly are exposed to many stresses. There are the physiological, related to decreased physical functional capacity and acute or chronic physical illness; there are the psychological, related to dependency, isolation, loneliness, inter- and intra- personal conflicts and intra-familial conflicts; and there are the sociological, involving personal and socioeconomic descriptions such as retirement, widowhood, loss of family and friends, and status upheaval. Under such stresses of loss, conflicts and tensions, symptoms of anxiety, depression, or somatic malfunction may develop.[32]

From the standpoint of geriatric pharmacology, it is a fact that drug use by the elderly has major economic and medical importance. In the mid-1970's they spent almost $100 for prescribed and over-the-counter drugs annually and averaged more than 13 prescriptions a year including renewals.[33] In 1974 the aged, who comprise 10 percent of our population, spent an estimated $2.3 billion on drugs and drug sundries. This was more than 20 percent of the total national drug bill. The per capita expenditure for prescribed drugs by the elderly exceeds that for all other age groups.

New Directions in Aging Research

The search for more knowledge about aging has intensified in recent years. This quest is important because our population is getting older. What are these older adults like physically and mentally? Even more crucial for the future is the question, what can be done to keep them healthy, active and productive? Scientists at the Gerontology Research Center in Baltimore, the intramural research facility of the National Institute on Aging, seek answers to these and other questions related to aging.[34]

The obvious need for tangible and immediate improvement in the quality of life for the aged has shifted research away from an exclusive disease orientation to a broader inquiry into normal physiological changes, the behavioral constitution of the aged, and the social, cultural and economic environment in which we grow old. These areas are investigated in the four branches and laboratories of the National Institute on Aging. Scientists at the Institute search for answers to the following questions.[35]

Clinical Physiology: What clinical, physiological or biomedical factors influence aging? Can the effects of disease be separated from those associated with growing older? Are there more accurate and efficient ways to identify early stages of disease in the elderly?

Behavioral Sciences: What are the behavioral changes that accompany aging? Is it possible to minimize losses in learning, memory and reasoning ability that occur in some older adults? Can visceral responses such as heart rhythm, blood pressure and sphincter activity be voluntarily controlled?

Molecular Aging: How do internal control mechanisms which regulate essential body functions fail with age? To what extent do changes with age in the genetic information systems influence aging? Can harmful changes found in cells of the aged be prevented, arrested or circumvented?

Cellular and Comparative Physiology: What age-related changes occur in dividing or nondividing cells of older organisms? Why do aged humans and animals experience losses of normal immune responses? To what degree can nutrition minimize changes in cellular metabolism and function during aging?

The accumulated expertise and excellent resources available at the National Institute on Aging's Baltimore facility make it ideally suited for research that will provide answers to the above questions.[36]

Research Studies in Dental Care for the Elderly

In 1972, the findings of a study indicated that it was difficult to motivate younger dentists and dental students to learn about the problems of the aged. It seemed that the dental schools did not give adequate attention to the masticatory function and acceptable dental esthetics for the aged patient.[37] However, in another study[38] done at the Harvard University School of Dental Medicine, students were provided with opportunities to function outside of the dental operatory. They demonstrated the needs of the chronically ill and how dentists could help in meeting these needs. The students used portable dental equipment to give such patients the benefit of dental care that they would normally not have had. A sample of 562 patients were selected from five nursing homes affiliated to a teaching hospital; 16 senior dental students worked with a dental assistant to give bedside treatment to the chronically ill. Of the patients screened, 41 percent were given dental treatment possible within the scope of the study, and cases that could not be treated within the scope of the program were referred to the nursing home dental consultant. Since the patients were in a variety of stages of severity of illness, the dental care given them was varied to suit individual needs, thus demonstrating to the students in a practical way the need for flexibility on the part of the dentist. Attention to the need for patience and sensitivity for the chronically ill was also stressed.

In a research project[39] dealing with dental care for the aged, it was argued that there is a general agreement among prosthodontists that the most difficult edentulous mouth to rehabilitate with complete dentures is the one in which the tissues cannot tolerate the presence of prosthesis. This condition may be due to systemic hormonal imbalance. Anabolic (constructive) sex hormones are necessary for health of the mucosa and bone, but since the secretions are reduced with advancing age, it is not uncommon to find that old people subject to postclimacteric syndrome cannot tolerate dentures even if they are technically perfect.

The immobility of the bedridden patients is responsible for a depletion of protein in the bone marrow and of calcium in the bone trabeculations. The end result is general bone loss, shifting of the mental foramen where nerves are easily exposed to denture pressure, causing severe pain. The author notes that the foregoing underscores the need for the dentist to bear in mind that "the success of any dental restoration or other prosthesis or appliance depends to a great extent on the environment in which it had to function." Such an environment may not be limited to the patient's mouth but to his or her home, work, city, world. He notes that the failure of many dentures is not because of faulty construction but because of the lack of basic biological knowledge of the tissues into which the prosthesis will be placed. A dentist who notices physical reasons why a denture would not be comfortable to use, should explain these to the patient before starting on constructon and must not fit a patient with a prosthesis first and then explain why later when the patient returns complaining of pain. It may be necessary, the author goes on, to construct a denture for a "sick" mouth, but the dentist owes it to both patient and family to state that the prosthesis should be used only for eating, and give instructions as to proper care of the dentures. A careful dentist will take all circumstances into consideration to decide whether a denture construction is contraindicated for certain edentulous people. If the dentist is convinced in such cases, a liquid but nutritious diet can be recommended.

It is important to note that within the past few years, several research studies have been done in dental care for the elderly in other societies. For example, the Proceedings of the Royal Society of Medicine[40] in 1973 indicated that people 60 and over who are dentate usually have about 16 teeth which are variously located to exhibit the skeleton of the dental cripple. In regard to the elderly patient, the author decries the attitude that treatment for such a patient should be of temporary or semipermanent nature, and he reminds the dentist about the variation among individuals and the fact that chronological age is a poor indicator of the way tissues behave in the face of dental intervention. Treating the elderly calls for two basic considerations: the physical condition and behavior of elderly tissues, and the neurological and psychological state of the patient. These, the author believes, will ensure adjustment of the treatment to the patient's adaptability; he gives suggestions about clinical procedures in varied dental health conditions of the aged.

Research[41] focusing upon the oral health needs in the elderly Danish population indicated that about 70 percent were edentulous in both jaws, and 80 percent in the maxilla, with a slightly larger percentage of women than men being edentulous. Partial dentures were common, while a large number of the subjects managed only with their few remaining natural teeth. The quality of the remaining natural teeth was examined and women were found to have better quality teeth than men. Clinical examination and evaluation of present dentures showed that some would need no treatment, since they were edentulous, but 75 percent of those still dentate needed full dentures. The main reason given for treatment by patients was faulty mastication.

An assessment of the oral mucosa, dentures, treatment

needs and habits indicated that the oral health of the elderly Danish population in the provincial areas was very poor and treatment needs extensive. The question is whether it is possible to motivate aged people to seek dental care when they are most often satisfied with their present dental state. The author concluded that is was the duty of the state to disseminate information to all old persons about the consequences of faulty dentures.

In 1974, another study[42] demonstrated that in a population where people live longer, the need for geriatric care increases, but it appears that adequate dental care for the elderly receives low priority. It is suggested that elderly dentists are more suited to treat the elderly because of the ripe experience of older practitioners and the common outlook they share with elderly patients, which make for attaining an overall good rapport.

That is not to say, the author cautions, that treating elderly patients should be the exclusive responsibility of the elderly dentists because such arrangements are not without danger; when the patient and dentist grow together, they share a common outlook, memories, and an emotional involvement with one another. The dentist may then be tempted to safeguard the patient and refrain from a treatment method that is thought likely to inconvenience the patient, whereas a younger and independent dentist might institute a more rigorous but necessary treatment.

The findings further indicated that management of the elderly patients is of two types, the technical and the psychological. A list is drawn up of the types of technical procedures that are more suited to the elderly patient during office visits; on the psychological level, the old person's feeling of helplessness and the inability to control day-to-day life events may be frustrating; such feelings should not be aggravated by the dentist. Some patients grow to a ripe age with minimal mental and physical impairment, but many more may be physically unpleasing and hard to cope with. Dentistry's obligation is more to the latter group, which deserves good understanding and constitutes more challenge to the dentist. To both the young and old dentists, the rule should be to honor one's father and mother in its widest social implications.

A research analysis in geriatric dentistry[43] points to the fact that there is a need not only for knowledge of clinical expertise but also for an awareness of social needs, preventive dentistry, and disorder both in thoughts and attitudes of the elderly. Thus, the practice of medicine and dentistry that is limited to reported needs will have an adverse effect on the elderly because few old people generally report their state of health. Thus, any delay until old people report or complain about their dental needs may be disastrous for them.

Preventive dentistry and preventive medicine are just as important for the elderly as for the young or middle-aged, hence periodic examinations must be insisted upon for the aged. This may not be an easy task, but arrangements can be made to identify those who are more vulnerable to deterioration and least likely to report—such as the aged who live alone: this group should be given a priority for care.

Nutrition is an important factor in the state of dental health of the aged. Connected with this are other factors such as food habits and attitudes that are actually psychological; loss of taste, which is physiologically linked; social circumstances, which throw light on the patterns of living and malnutrition; and living alone, which often affects adversely the availability and consumption of a balanced diet. In these areas, community intervention is very essential.

The study provides several technical suggestions to be implemented in treating old people in the areas of diagnoses, use of dental chair and oral medicine, oral rehabilitation, dental therapeutics and prosthetic care. Emphasis is placed upon the importance of maintaining rapport between the dentist and patient, development of a thorough medical and social history of the patient and domiciliary visits to the elderly by dentists.

An evaluation of the attitudes of a group of elderly edentulous patients toward dentists, dentures, and dentistry was carried out in England.[44] The sample study consisted of 286 men and 414 women; they were of reasonable mental and physical health whose ages averaged 62 and ranged from 18 to 89; the bulk of the population (69 percent) consisted of persons over 60, predominantly of low socioeconomic and educational levels and living on pensions but attending institutional establishments for their medical and dental needs.

The respondents were interviewed about their attendance at the dental clinic, how and why they became edentulous, their attitude to restorative work, and their denture experience. The results were as follows. The average length of time since the last visit to a dentist was about 6.4 years; most patients felt it necessary to see a dentist only if they had any discomfort with their dentures. The reasons given for visiting the dentists varied: two most frequently mentioned were ill-fitting dentures and broken or lost dentures; other reasons were that the dentures caused pain, and sometimes resulted in an unsatisfactory poor appearance. The older patients were generally less satisfied; for those over 60, physiological changes in bone and oral mucosa common among long-time denture wearers were found. When asked why they had their teeth extracted and how they felt in general with natural teeth, most members of the study sampled cited caries as the cause of the loss of their teeth; they had refused partial dentures and preferred their remaining teeth be extracted since they felt they would lose them sooner or later anyway.

The findings further suggested that little or no attempt had been made by the dentists to instruct patients about the maintenance of the health of the oral tissues or in the use of their dentures. The elderly patients in the sample considered natural teeth to be unreliable, uncomfortable and painful so that they were not reluctant to have them extracted. These pateints saw their dentist as one who was mechanically inclined, that is, removing teeth and constructing dentures.

It seemed that these attitudes might have arisen because dentistry, like surgery, was perceived as something that brought imaginary threat of injury; thus, it produced fear and resentment on the part of the public. Such perception of dentistry, the author cautioned, was dependent on the social, economic, and educational level of each patient; he then listed types of attitudes common among all age-sex groups, together with reasons behind such attitudes. The conclusion was that serious communication between dentist and patient was lacking; a solution would be to teach dentists to communicate more effectively with their patients.

A dental survey[45] was done in Wales to examine the dental needs of old people who were 65 years old and confined to home and institutions. The purpose of the research was to consider ways by which these old people could be ensured continued dental care; they were, therefore, given a questionnaire and a clinical examination.

Sixty-five percent of the respondents were found to be wearing complete dentures, and of these, 33 percent had inadequate dentures; 41 percent of all sampled had not seen a dentist for over 20 years; a few had experienced unusual oral sensations and temporary taste impairment. In general, the type of service found to be needed was prosthetic and oral health education. Many dentures were found to be dirty; more men than women were found to have poor oral hygiene; cracked, ill-fitting or broken dentures had not been satisfactorily adjusted or repaired before the study.

The findings further indicated that for long-term treatment, management and finance, dentists ought to visit old people's homes, using mobile and specially equipped vehicles, or have the patients brought by car or ambulance to the nearest treatment center. They stressed the need for community dental health service, but before such facilities are available, limited service should be provided by a dental hospital to this special class of patients in the community.

Along similar lines of analysis, a report of dental findings in a survey of geriatric patients in England reveals some interesting results.[46] The study sample consisted of 300 subjects who were both out- and inpatients of a university college dental school, and assessed dental needs for treatment in a group of elderly people in London, and how treatment for them could be achieved.

The average age of the subjects was 70.5 years; they were of varied socioeconomic backgrounds. Most of the outpatients were ambulant, but 60 percent of the inpatients were bedridden; senility and mental deterioration were among the chief reasons for those hospitalized.

The findings showed that 30 percent of the outpatients and 20 percent of the inpatients still had some of their teeth present. Periodontal disease was rife, probably because of substandard oral hygiene; many of the retained teeth were severely abraded, and half of these patients needed tooth restorations and periodontal care. Between 50 and 75 percent of dentures worn were considered by both patients and dentists to be unsatisfactory because of poor retention or instability of the appliances. The general standard of denture hygiene was poor, and dentures were the chief source of pain experienced by these patients.

Of the 300 patients, 206 were edentulous; out of this group, 11 percent had no dentures at all. About half of those edentulous complained of denture pain and discomfort. One reason was the excessive age of the dentures, over a third being 10 years old or more. Oral pathologic and radiographic examinations were done. About 49 percent of all patients showed pathologic signs that needed further investigations.

Modern medicine, the report asserted, aimed not only at prolonging life for a greater number of people but also at improving the quality of such life; oral health and the standard of dental appliances worn ought therefore be as good as possible. It was pointed out that one had to distinguish between statistical need for treatment as shown by the survey, and the realistic necessity for treatment feasible to be carried out. Although the research demonstrated extensive need for complete dentures, it also showed that some of the cases, being extremely difficult, would need a specialist's treatment, while about 50 percent of all inpatients' dental problems were so complicated that it would be almost impractical to give them any treatment at all.

The findings also stressed the importance of the involvement of local authorities in supplying a community dental health service to provide care for the elderly and for the young. Plans for dental care of the aged must be taken into account as various reorganizations of health and welfare services were being done.

From the perspective of dietary selection by elderly persons, another study[47] examined the effects of various diets on the state of dental health of a sample of pensioners. A stratified sample by age and sex of 75 pensioners in Portsmouth, England, had received meals on wheels and they were later selected for the pilot survey. The respondents were interviewed by a home economist regarding their food habits, especially their hard and soft foods, and a dental examination was later performed by the dentist. The findings showed that the dental state of most of the subjects was poor; two-thirds of the dentures examined were of such poor quality that some of those who were edentulous used their dentures part of the time or not at all for chewing. These conditions were also reflected in the restricted food selection of the subjects. The study emphasized that a more careful examination ought to be made concerning the dental needs of housebound elderly persons.

By contrast, research done in geriatric care in Israel[48] reported more favorable conditions for the aged. They have the opportunity to live in separate communities. Health care is provided by nurses who are young and specially trained for this purpose. These nurses can request the services of a dentist or physician whenever the need arises. The health care system for the aged seems to function well.

Chapter 10

Social Change and Dental Care

At any given moment in time, the social structure or framework of a society may appear to be a static entity; but viewed over a long period of time, the structure can be seen to be a dynamic organization of components, each changing internally, growing or decaying and in an everchanging relationship with all the other components.

Behavioral scientists often use the two terms, social change and cultural change, interchangeably and at times substitute the term "sociocultural change" to include both kinds of changes. In brief, social change is a continuous process of variation in social behavior which is present in all societies, as in all other forms of modifications in life. It refers to alterations in social structures. Of particular interest are those social changes that have relatively important consequences and that tend to be comparatively long standing.

In the *Gemeinschaft*, change is rather slow; as each generation succeeds its predecessor, it is fitted into the positions left vacant. Life continues in very much the same way over a period of many generations. Small changes do, of course, occur in all societies and not even people with rural attitudes and values have remained unchanged from the early days of the human race. In the *Gesellschaft*, change is most rapid and dynamic due to the high degree of industrialization, invention, discovery and the diffusion of ideas.

Causes of Social Change

With the inception of the Industrial Revolution, the speed

of social change has increased continuously in Western societies. This change has spread to almost every part of the world and has affected both developing and developed nations to varying degrees. Some of the factors affecting the rate of change are as follows:

The Physical Environment—Changes in the physical environment may come about very slowly and may be very difficult to observe. Nevertheless, they may present a challenge to people in a society in such a way that some adjustment would have to be made to meet the new conditions of life, just as, for example, the migration of a large group of people to a different environment produces many changes in a culture.

Population Change—Any major change in the size or distribution of a population always produces social changes. An increased population in a society may result in migration or improved production which brings about social change.

Technological and Economic Factors—Inventions and innovations may have a far-reaching impact on the social structure of a society.

Isolation and Contact—Societies with the greatest contact on a national and international level usually demonstrate a very high rate of change. Societies that are isolated tend to limit intercultural relations and as a result show a very low rate of social change.

The Structure of a Society and Culture—If a society is tightly structured, as it is in India, then social change would be rather expensive and difficult to introduce.

Perceived Needs—A society's recognition of a need is a prerequsite for social change.

Cultural Factors—Not all elements of a society change at the same rate of speed. The structures of the major institutions change more slowly. People's values, on the other hand, are so deeply incorporated into the personality that the rate of change is often unnoticed. This disparity in the rates of change among the different elements of a society is called *cultural lag*. William F. Ogburn was the first person to coin the term. He distinguished between the "material" and "nonmaterial" aspects of culture. Changes in the material culture stimulate changes in the nonmaterial culture, but the nonmaterial is slow to adapt itself to changes in the material and this gives rise to a "lag" between the two aspects.

The above aspects of social change in a society are closely interrelated and changes in any one lead ultimately to changes in the others. For example, changes in the density of population are responsible for many changes in the social organization of a society. As the density of a population increases, one may expect that the division of labor and specialization may also increase. If these changes occur, then they affect the economic institution as well. The pressure of population growth may in favorable situations stimulate invention and economic growth. On the other hand, changes in the structures of the health care institution and the growth of medical knowledge may be a factor in population growth by decreasing the death rate of a society. We shall now consider a few selected theories of social change.

Theories of Social Change

Two recent theories that are essentially psychological in nature are those of David C. McClelland[1] and Everett E. Hagen.[2] McClelland attributed change to the growth in numbers of individuals who have high "n-ach" (need for achievement). He demonstrated a method of measuring the individual's need for achievement from his creative writing. He became interested in the causes of economic development and in the relationship between these and the level of the need for achievement.

McClelland, assuming that a high level of "n-ach" would stimulate economic growth of a society, attempted to measure the relationship between the variables. He measured the level of "n-ach" in a society by the interpretation of the amount of achievement imagery in the stories written for children. He then compared this with the subsequent economic growth (measured in units of electricity produced) and discovered a statistical relationship between the two variables. Although an "n-ach" could be analyzed by the content of children's stories, the fundamental cause in an increase in "n-ach" was to be found in the parents' attitudes toward their children—in other words, in child care methods.

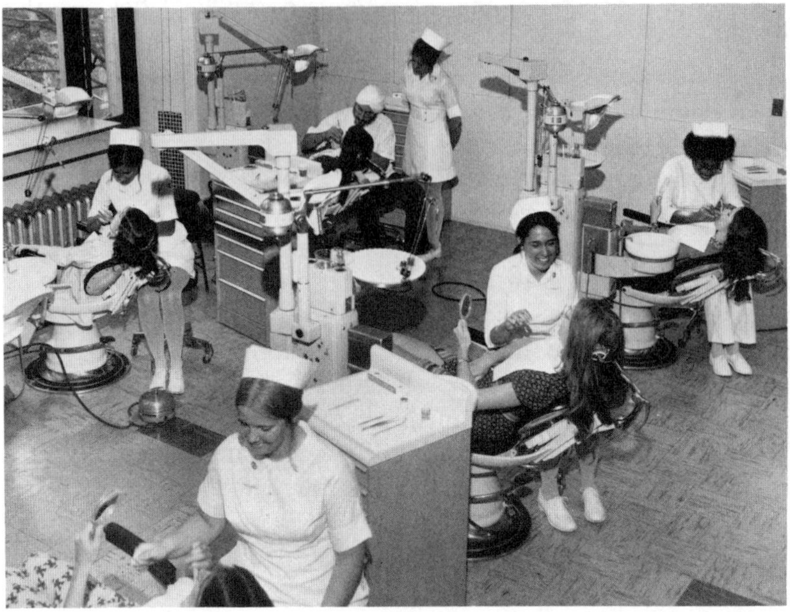

Dental hygiene students in clinical training (photograph by Ralph R. Lobene)

Hagen's views about social change in society are similar to those of McClelland. Both see the source of personality type in this kind of child rearing practiced within a society. He emphasizes the importance of creative personalities. For example, Hagen argues that the innovators in various societies were people who had experienced fears of status deprivation. They were the sons of fathers whose position in society was being threatened and who could not give the sons an adequate role model.

Other theorists who contributed to the various forms of special change in society include Ralf Dahrendorf and Karl Marx, proponents of the conflict theory. Max Weber attempted to show that ideas are necessary though not sufficient causes of change, while Talcott Parsons and Gerhard Lenski proposed new evolutionary theories of social change.

Social Change and Health Care

From the point of view of the health care institutions in

the United States, within recent years a tremendous change has occurred in the sheer number of patients discharged from short-stay hospitals. Data indicate that a substantial portion of the increase in hospital use can be explained by the increased use among persons 45 years of age and over, especially those 65 years of age and over. Further "about 13 percent of the estimated 22.8 million discharges during July 1962-June 1963 were among persons 65 years of age and over, compared with 18 percent of the estimated 29.3 million discharges during 1974. The increase in hospitalization utilization among persons in the older age group apparently reflects the influence of the medicare program in July, 1966."[3]

Within recent years, various changes have occurred in the number, size and ownership of nursing homes. In 1973, there were 21,834 nursing homes in the United States. These homes contained 1,327,704 beds, an average of 61 beds per home. This average bed capacity showed an increase over the 1971 average and continued the trend of increasing bed capacities since 1967. Between 1971 and 1973, there was a decrease of more than 1,100 homes for homes with under fifty beds and an increase of almost 950 for those with fifty or more beds.[4]

Observations reveal two types of nursing homes—nursing care homes and personal care and other homes. Between 1967 and 1973, nursing care homes showed a substantial increase, while personal care homes and others showed increases and decreases during the same period.[5]

Over the past years, changes had resulted in the number and utilization of speciality hospitals such as psychiatric, rehabilitation, chronic disease and tuberculosis. For example, rehabilitation hospitals showed an increase from 1971 through 1973. The average bed capacity for psychiatric hospitals decreased from 785 to 666, and for tuberculosis hospitals it decreased from 180 to 157. Although chronic disease hospitals decreased in numbers, their bed capacities increased from 273 to 319. Rehabilitation hospitals increased their numbers and at the same time expanded their bed capacities.[6] The occupancy rates for these four types of hospitals remained relatively consistent for the two years, whereas the turnover rates (admissions per bed) particularly for tuberculosis hospitals, had remarkable changes.

Thus, the number of admissions per bed in tuberculosis hospitals went from 2.0 in 1971 to 2.5 in 1973, a 25 percent increase.[7]

Changes occurred in health facilities other than hospitals and nursing homes. The "other health facilities" included resident schools or homes for the deaf, the blind, the physically handicapped, the mentally retarded, the emotionally disturbed, unwed mothers, dependent children (and orphans), and alcoholics or drug abusers. Data show that most of these other facilities experienced a decline in bed capacity from 1971 to 1973. The bed capacity for unwed mothers and emotionally disturbed individuals increased to some extent. The occupancy rates suggest that very little change took place over the two year period, and these changes were in the form of decreases.[8]

Changes in the health care institution as a whole, be it in hospitals, nursing homes, clinics, or in the physician's office, do affect the dental care of a population. The modern profession of dentistry plays an important role in a changing society. As society changes, people take on new responsibilities for health, masticatory function, and esthetics. Many individuals anticipate future dental problems and seek to have them treated at an early stage. Indeed, modern dentistry has convinced the public that an edentulous mouth is a less than ideal condition and is not a necessary result of age. Furthermore, many individuals are now aware of the fact that neglect of any tooth may result in lack of function, discomfort and loss, and ultimately lead to prosthetics.[9]

Research Studies in Social Change and Dental Care

Society granted the health professions special rights and privileges, hence these professions especially must be responsive to the society's needs at all times. As the needs of society change, so also must the profession learn to adapt itself to the new needs accompanying such change, as indicated by a recent study.[10]

The study notes one of society's changes, namely the shift in attitude toward health services as dramatized by the enactment of Medicare and Medicaid. This shift signaled the trend toward the recognition that health care was a right, not a privilege, and the profession of dentistry must take account of this attitude. The study suggested that dentistry had been attempting to meet both its patients' and society's needs over the years through its educational instructions.

In the 1960's emphasis was placed on the need by dentists for social awareness; this was necessary because the majority of dentists came from the middle and upper classes and these individuals were mostly white. Since such recruitment was restrictive, it was difficult to expose dentists to the population as a whole, and to study the characteristics and attitudes of patients who were from lower classes and of minority ethnic groups. These disadvantaged groups usually had lower incomes and restricted access to dental care. This lack of awareness made it impossible for the dentist to organize a practice in order to take account of these other groups and hence the profession was restricted in its ability to serve a wider spectrum of the population.

The traditional practice which made dental service available only to those with the proper interest, motivation, and financial resources must give way to providing services to all. Since the community was having an increased number of agencies and programs which provided health services for the people, and Congress was likely to come up sooner or later with a form of national health insurance, the study suggested that the profession needed a sophisticated awareness of these trends in organized health care and should anticipate methods to reduce problems of cost and delivery of care; these would help the profession to respond intelligently to Congressional action in financing health services.

It was suggested in this report that the social awareness of the 1960's should be followed by skillful social action to meet the problems that would come up during the 1970's and 1980's. The dental profession must be prepared to be an agent of change, moving ahead of the population and the politicians by initiating new programs, and should insist that such programs be implemented; it must be actively involved in maintaining these new strategies and evaluating the new operations.

The dentistry community must find ways to deliver programs for those who were usually shut out of them; consumers of dental service must be involved in planning such service since the expert knowledge of dentists is mainly technical and does not mean that they have all the answers to planning and implementing all dental services. Consumer involvement and participation, therefore, was necessary in all aspects of health care, including preventive, educational, and curative programs.

The author suggested that to bring oral health within the reach of everyone who needed it, dental manpower must be increased for the next fifteen years. Many aspects of practice, professional examinations and licensure procedures that are out of date, hence restricting the number of new dentists, must be revamped; the use of auxiliaries must be increased and the dentists must be redistributed to make service available to areas in dire need of dentists. The quality of care becomes important, especially since unions or governments would pay for dental service; thus the profession must devise ways to monitor dental care provided by dentists.

In the past, the profession was largely concerned with individual restoration, but for the present and the future, a new orientation of health care is needed. The scope of care must be broadened to include the entire mouth and the total care of the individual. Though some progress has been made in the past several decades still the maintenance of sound dentition in a sound body must continuously be made the goal of dental care. The traditional one-to-one basis of private practice should provide no satisfaction to a dentist who realizes the need for rehabilitation of a host of others in the community who are not receiving care. The dentist must learn new skills in leadership and management, for these are needed whenever he or she is called upon to assume more and more responsibility in community dental care, a role which the public health dentists used to play in the past.

In the 1973 presidential address of the American Association of Orthodontists at Dallas, Dr. Hubert J. Bell discussed a meeting of internists to which he was invited, reporting that most of the findings centered on socioeconomic problems facing the nation and the frequent question about why the physicians, having been loved and respected over the years, suddenly began to lose the respect and incur instead the resentment of the people. He suggested that the rapid changes taking place probably made some professional persons lose their humanity in their dealings with the people, and called attention to the impression held by many people that the health professionals treated them like commodities and as if they were just as expendable.[11]

Dr. Bell believed that what was happening to medicine might soon start to happen to dentistry. His main interest was in preserving the status quo for dentistry from the encroachment of its rights by government intervention. He felt that the best deterrent to the socioeconomic health proposals of government was to keep the patients satisfied and not make them feel like objects. This, he belived, would create an image that would delay such government intervention for years to come. It was his view that policy makers in government knew very little and yet were prepared to tell dentists what to do; it was his aim that dentistry, with all of its human and other resources, should survive the trends for change.

In a somewhat similar vein, Dr. Kenneth V. Randolph noted at the Annual Meeting of the American College of Dental Examiners how the role of dental examiners was affected by a changing society.[12] He pointed out that the most important task performed by the college was in providing assurance to lay persons that dental care quality control was being provided to the society by certifying the all around competence of dentists released to practice in the society.

He stressed the need for study by the profession of how best the society could be served; he pointed out the increasing demands for dental care, and among the reasons given for this increase was that the stigma of pain associated with a dental office was decreasing, while socioeconomic factors no longer meant that only the affluent could get care. He did not think, however, that good dental care was yet within reach of everyone: for one thing, the dentist-population ratio was still unfavorable; this was worsened by the increased longevity of many people, which meant that more people would be needing dental care over longer years. Many studies, he found, supported the need for more dentists, and he asserted that dental educators, examiners, and practitioners must take appropriate steps so that the profession could meet its responsibilities.

He noted that dentistry had been unreceptive to government intervention, but he believed that some accommodation between the federal government and dentists at the state level must be made so as to achieve a resolution of the problem. It was suggested that two years of compulsory assignment to areas in dire need of dentists could substitute for the two-year military service demanded at that time by the government. With the increase of various types of insurance programs, he predicted that more lay agencies would become involved with health programs; thus the profession must observe such changes cautiously and the examiners were urged to play a leading role.

The changes toward more liberal views that challenged the family, home and morality of the nation had not spared health professions, Dr. Randolph continued; this was evidenced by various revolutionary opinions and philosophies embraced by students and members of the faculty alike. He cautioned that the dental examiners should not be surprised to find that their position was challenged since they were representing an authority; however, since they were the protectors of the public in the areas of dental care, they must be alert to these changes.

In an attempt to predict what the future role of the dentist would look like, Dr. Randolph suggested that the dentists of 1985 would be sort of super diagnosticians and planners; they would be directing a supporting staff and their work would be similar to that of business persons. He believed that dentists were not going to abdicate their traditional roles, which had historically given dentistry its current image. Supervising dental clinical work rather than performing it could in no way make the average dentist proud and satisfied with the profession.

On the role of auxiliaries, he believed that the profession should isolate these tasks that must be performed by the dentist and no one else; this would help, he believed, to silence the uneasiness felt by many dentists about their future roles. He felt that delivery of health services could gain a lot by expanding duties performed by auxiliaries provided they were properly supervised. Dr. Randolph finally called attention to the long historical process through which dentistry had developed to its present status and noted that changes improperly thought out could reverse the progress made in traditional dental care. He also emphasized the need for more preventive dentistry and urged continuing education for dentists.

Writing on social attitudes toward dental care, Hillenbrand[13] identified two major changes that had occurred in such attitudes. First was the fact that dental care no longer concerned mere absence of illness but involved the idea of total well-being as pointed out by the World Health Organization. Second was the view that both dental and total health were not the privilege of the few who had the financial means but the right of the many. These two ideas, Hillenbrand said, embraced the problem of health services delivery which beset all countries of the world, regardless of the health resources available to each.

Among the causes for the changing social attitudes toward dental health noted were the rising expectation of people in all societies for a better life and better health, the increased use of governmental funds to finance dental care, and better education about oral health by the mass media. National governments all over the world had also been influenced by the various W.H.O. programs in the areas of health, which led to eradication of many of the communicable diseases, and by the Federation Dentaire Internationale (FDI), which had been playing a role similar to that of W.H.O. in the areas of dental health. The FDI once brought 60 national associations together for an exchange of information on dental health and urged them to raise the standard of dental health in their various countries.

Hillenbrand then suggested factors which had influenced a greater awareness of dental health, among which were fluoridation, increasingly accepted as a preventive rather than curative dentistry; the concept of a dental health delivery system that organized resources and brought dental care within the reach of individuals; the introduction of modern techniques in dentistry, which had reduced public fear of pain associated with dental works; the advent of dental education incorporating the concepts of social and behavioral sciences, thereby making dentists more sensitive to patients' other needs and motivation for seeking care; the use of dental auxiliaries, which helped to change people's attitude to dental care because these auxiliaries had more time to instruct patients than did the dentist; and the development of various payment plans enabling patients with modest means to seek care.

Poupard,[14] writing on the future roles of dental

auxiliaries, also noted the increase in the number of people seeking oral health care, and the reasons citied were similar to some of those already suggested by Hillenbrand. Because of this growing awareness of oral health, however, Poupard felt that demand would rise for more comprehensive care and better preventive diagnostic techniques, together with supportive and rehabilitative care. The new legislation expanding health insurance coverage, encouraging more and more people to want the best of oral care, might in the end prove frustrating if adequate provision for the desired services was not made. The problem in providing such adequate services would not be solved by merely increasing the number of dentists. The major solution suggested was to increase the number of professionally trained auxiliaries. It was recommended that full use of the dental team, consisting of the dentist, dental artisan and dental hygienist, should be an everyday part of the dental delivery system. The dental laboratory technicians who were usually trained on the job should also be trained in the junior and community college programs and at the vocational high schools. The dental aides could be trained at vocational schools or on-the-job. The dental assistants, with critical selection in recruitment, could be trained to perform certain technical procedures.

Among dental auxiliaries, the dental hygienist is seen as a well-trained professional capable of certain important functions and decision-making. Poupard believed that the role of the hygienists could be increased in the disciplines of periodontal disease and oral pathology, in addition to the curative and management assignments they are usually given. It was suggested that both the hygienist and dental artisan should be encouraged in upward mobility by providing access to the baccalaureate degree for those qualified and willing to train.

A study forecasting a future shock for dentistry is that of Weinberg,[15] who felt that the profession was not keeping pace with the rapid new changes taking place within the society, with the main culprit being change itself. He noted that changes were taking place in education, therapy, practice and in payment for care. He recognized that the demands these changes would make on dentists would differ; some dentists would readily adjust, while others might give up and drop out of practice.

Changes in dental school education which he noted included new and more flexible curricula, giving these schools an opportunity to experiment with new courses. Such changes, however, would create problems for students who would no longer be able to predictably track courses from one year to another. Many of these students would find after graduation that the emphasis on prevention was changing society's perception of good dentistry and that substandard treatment would no longer be accepted. Because of increased use of fluoridation, the incidence of decayed teeth among the youth would decrease. By the end of the century, expanded functions of auxiliaries might include placing, carving or polishing filling materials in dentist-prepared cavities as well as doing more complicated work than is now being assigned to them. A better educated public and better financial resources would mean that the dentist would have a larger part of the population and a greater number of younger people to treat; because of the new financial resources to pay for care, more of the dentist's income would be derived from third party payments. Weinberg believed that these changes might result in painful adaptive experiences for some dentists because they were ill-prepared by their education and experience to face and accept change. While some would be unable to function in the ensuing social flux, he hoped that the majority of dentists would.

Another writer calling for action now in order to forestall future shock was Rickles.[16] Noting pressures mounting within the society for changes in dentistry, he suggested that there must be a move toward a future that would be acceptable if not loved by the profession, so long as it could meet the increasing expectations of the public. He warned that if the professions hope to continue their future self-determination with minimal risks, they must look ahead.

In addition to the usual appeal for better education and utilization of auxiliaries, Rickles made more provocative suggestions for the dentists themselves. He believed that society would demand that the leader of the oral health team be as competent as any other health specialist. Since auxiliaries would increasingly be used to perform most of the technical procedures, the dentist could then become this leader. The resistance of many dentists to increased use of dental auxiliaries, he felt, was traceable to a sense of uneasiness on the part of many dentists concerning this new leadership role. A statement by a dean of the Harvard School of Dental Medicine supports this contention: that is, "the dentist of today is overtrained for what he does and undertrained for what he should be doing." In the dean's view dentists did not need to devote much time to the study of the basic sciences because they did not use pertinent parts of them, being more concerned with mechnical restorative aspects of practice.

For restorative practice, therefore, Rickles felt that dentists were overtrained in the basic sciences. However, they did not have enough training in biomedical areas to be able to evaluate the total patient, a concept that was paid only lip service both in the dental school and in practice. In picturing what the dentists of the future would be, Rickles saw them retaining technical competency and being better able to coordinate and direct the activities of the auxiliary personnel. They would also be more sensitive to the problems of the society.

The evaluation and management of the patient's nondental oral diseases would be another asset of the dentist of the future. In his opinion, at present neither dentists nor physicians are adequately trained in the prevention, diagnosis and treatment of oral cancer and other oral lesions. Many in both professions are unfamiliar with the manifestations of systemic diseases. Furthermore, most dentists are ill prepared to manage patients who suffer from known conditions such as diabetes, hypertension or cardiovascular or kidney disease, or to properly consider the effect of medications being given for systemic diseases on the treatment of oral diseases. Rickles believed that the dentist of the future would be able to better manage the oral conditions of patients with known diseases. The dentists of today, according to Rickles, were in the unenviable position of carrying out procedures that were potentially harmful to patients because they lacked training that would alert them to such conditions. This was the type of situation that could and often did cause friction between physicians and dentists on the question of equality of hospital privileges for the two professions.

Rickles felt that the training of general dentists to perform surgery and prescribe drugs was inadequate because they could cause iatrogenic harm to their patients. In Europe, there were two levels of practitioners engaged in oral care: the dental mechanics and the stomatologists or physicians who were concerned mainly with medical and surgical problems of the mouth. He wanted to see dentists well trained in internal medicine and emergency care so they would be able to manage, or at least be aware of, the suspected or unsuspected systemic diseases of their patients; the dentists could then choose to have additional training in one of the specialties such as orthodontics, oral surgery, or oral pathology.

Concluding, Rickles believed that the potential of over 100,000 dentists in the country for finding early systemic diseases was great, given the proper education. The suitability of dentists was even greater in this area since their patients with such diseases were likely to visit the dentist while relatively well, whereas they would seek a physician when they were really sick. He suggested experimental education along the lines already stated for undergraduate training of dentists, as well as continuing education for dentists already in practice. Similarly upgraded educational training was suggested for auxiliaries.

Insight to the future of dentistry and the delivery of dental care can be found in an unusual editorial appearing in a dental journal.[17]

> To refuse to see that great changes are at hand, as concerns the standing and practice of the dental professions, is simply to shut one's eyes. Of no one thing are we more assured than that dentistry of today must either advance or give place: to attempt to confine it to its present limits is to seek to control that progress which is itself evolution.

That advice to dentistry was unusual only in that it was published in 1872. It was as true then as it is now. The total dental community must be prepared to change and this change must begin with the education of the dentist—the person who is to assume the responsibility for directing the oral health team of the future.

A concept of the future dental practitioner was described by Lobene[18] as one who would be biologically based, clinically competent, socially sensitive and community oriented. In addition, this future practitioner must be a manager capable of directing the activities of many auxiliaries if the delivery of care is to be cost effective. The fact that a dentist can direct the activities of multiple operating auxiliaries has been demonstrated in a recent study of the use of advanced-skills hygienists to provide restorative services.[19] This study also predicted that the use of these auxiliaries, as was done in a private practice simulation, could reduce the cost of care to the consumer or third party payer.

The future practitioner will bear little resemblance to the dentist of today. This new breed will know more oral medicine and medicine, although they will not be required to have a comprehensive knowledge of the practice of medicine. They will administer many new diagnostic tests for the detection of precarious lesions and subclinical periodontal diseases. Great attention will focus on the detection of oral cancer and hypertension, with referral to appropriate specialists for treatment.

In the twenty-first century, this new dentist will become a stomatologist and delegate many of the mechanical, repetitive, reversible procedures to auxiliaries working under supervision. In this capacity, the biological base of the stomatologist will need to be broad in order to make the judgments necessary to delegation. Delegation of traditional dentists' functions to appropriately educated and trained expanded-functions auxiliaries is the key to high quality and cost effective care for the consumer, as well as being the rationale for the development of the stomatologist. Organized dentistry, government, the public, researchers and dental teachers must work together to foster this advancement to the age of stomatology while surrendering the mechanical aspects of dental therapy to the technicians.

References

Chapter 1

[1]Gordon C. Zahn, *What Is Society?* (New York: Hawthorn Books, 1964), p. 36.

[2]Ralph Linton, *Culture and Mental Disorders* (Springfield, Ill.: Charles C. Thomas, 1956), pp. 4-44.

[3]Reece McGee, *Points of Departure: Basic Concepts in Sociology* (Hinsdale, Ill.: Dryden Press, 1975), p. 35.

[4]*Ibid.*

[5]James Skipper and Emily Mumford, *Sociology in Hospital Care* (New York: Harper & Row, 1967), p. 28.

[6]L. Saunders, *Cultural Differences and Medical Care* (New York: Russell Sage Foundation, 1954).

[7]Barry H. Grayson, Paul Van Niewerbugh, and Samuel Dworkin, "Culture and Caries," *New York State Dental Journal* **38** (January 1972):15-22.

[8]*Ibid.*

[9]Mark Zborowski, *People in Pain* (San Francisco: Jossey-Bass, 1969).

[10]Gordon Allport, "Perception and Public Health," in *Health and the Community*, ed. Alfred H. Katz and Jean Spencer Felton (New York: Free Press, 1965), p. 501.

[11]T.A. Gonda, "The Relation Between Complaints of Persistent Pain and Family Size," *Journal of Neurology, Neurosurgery, and Psychiatry* **25** (August 1962):277-81.

[12]Skipper and Mumford, *Sociology in Hospital Care*, p. 136.

[13]Earl Lomon Koos, *The Health of Regionville: What the People Thought and Did About It* (New York: Columbia University Press, 1954).

[14]James W. Vander Zanden, *Sociology: A Systematic Approach* (New York: Ronald Press, 1970), p. 57.

[15]Robert Bierstedt, *The Social Order* (New York: McGraw-Hill, 1974), p. 221.

[16]Louis Wirth, *The Ghetto* (Chicago: University of Chicago Press, 1928).

[17]Mark Lisagor and Donald L. Rowland, "The UCLA-Whiteriver Dental Project," *Journal of Public Health Dentistry* **34** (Spring 1974):94-103.

[18]R. Dan Corry and Louis F. Cannavale, "Expanded Functions Training for Dental Assistants in the Indian Health Service," *Journal of the American Dental Association* **85** (December 1972):1343-8.

[19]A.L. Heise, "Meeting the Dental Treatment Needs of Indigent Rural Children," *Health Services Reports* **88** (August-September 1973):591-660.

[20]A.S.T. Franks and G.B. Winter, "Management of the Handicapped and Chronic Sick Patient in the Dental Practice," *British Dental Journal* **136** (January 1974):20-3.

[21]Joseph L. Dicks, "Effects of Different Communication Techniques on the Cooperation of the Mentally Retarded Child During Dental Procedure," *Journal of Dentistry for Children* **41** (July-August 1974):283-8.

[22]Richard H. Gordon, "Meeting Dental Needs of the Aged," *American Journal of Public Health* **62** (March 1972):385-8.

[23]H. Erke, "The Dentist-Patient Relationship: A Psychological View," *Öffentliche Gesundheitswesen* **33** (March 1971):13-21.

[24]S.F. Parkin, J.A. Hargraves and Joan Weuman, "Children's Dentistry in General Practice, II – Management of Children in Dental Surgery," *British Dental Journal* **129** (July 1970):83-5.

[25]M.A. Lubespere, "The Psychology of the Dental Patient," *Revue Odontostomatologie du Midi de la France* **28** (3d qtr 1970):155-73.

[26]G. Koch and T. Martinsson, "Socio-ondontologic Investigation of School Children with High and Low Caries Frequency, I – Socio-economic Background," *Odontologisk Revy* (Malmö) **21** (1970):207-8.

[27]Josef Wodniecki, "Practical Measures for the Prevention of Oral Diseases," *Czasopismo Stomatologiczne* **23** (June 1970):643-7.

Chapter 2

[1]Rene Dubos, *Man Adapting* (New Haven, Conn.: Yale University Press, 1971), pp. 348-9.

[2]H. B. Richardson, *Patients Have Families* (New York: Commonwealth Fund, 1948), p. 76.

[3]Theordore K. Selkirk, "Hereditary Dark Teeth," *Journal of Pediatrics* **46** (February 1955):192-9.

[4]Talcott Parsons, *The Social System* (Glencoe, Ill.: Free Press, 1951), pp. 436-7. See also his restatement in his article "Definitions of Health and Illness in the Light of American Values and Social Structure," in *Patients, Physicians and Illness*, 2d ed., ed. E. Gartly Jaco (New York: Free Press, 1972), pp. 117-8.

[5]M.V. Susser and W. Watson, *Sociology in Medicine* (London: Oxford University Press, 1971), p. 281.

[6]U.S. Department of Health, Education and Welfare, Public Health Service, *Periodontal Disease among Youths 12-17 Years United States* (Washington, D.C.: U.S. Gov. Printing Office, 1974), p. 5.

[7]*Ibid.*, p. 7.

[8]U.S. Department of Health, Education, and Welfare, Public Health Service, *Decayed, Missing, and Filled Teeth among Youths 12-17 Years United States* (Washington, D.C.: U.S. Gov. Printing Office, 1974), p. 7.

[9]U.S. Department of Health, Education and Welfare, Public Health

Service, *Oral Hygiene among Youths 12-17 Years United States* (Washington, D.C.: U.S. Gov. Printing Office, 1975), p. 5.

[10]Sharon Brooks and Robert A. Bagramian, "Project Head Start—A Dental Public Health Apprentice," *Journal of the Michigan Dental Association* **53** (July-August 1971):232-4.

[11]Chester W. Douglas and Dennis C. Stacey, "The Clinic Habit: A Sociological Analysis of a Dental Public Health Program," *Journal of Public Health Dentistry* **33** (Winter 1973):56-8.

[12]Sheldon D. Rose, "Group Training of Parents as Behavior Modifers," *Social Work* **19** (March 1974):156-62.

[13]Editorial, "Dental Caries," *South African Medical Journal* **47** (February 1973):202.

[14]Pitirim A. Sorokin, *The Crisis of Our Age* (New York: Dutton, 1942), p. 167.

[15]William J. Goode, *The Family* (Englewood Cliffs, N. J.: Prentice-Hall, 1964), p. 92.

[16]Robert J. Haggerty and Joel J. Alpert, "The Child, His Family, and Illness," *Postgraduate Medicine* **34** (September 1963):228-9.

[17]*Ibid.*

[18]Joel J. Alpert, "The Functions of the Family Physical," *Connecticut Medicine* **32** (September 1968):664.

[19]John F. Neuman and Odin W. Anderson, *Patterns of Dental Science Utilization in the United States: A Nationwide Survey* (Chicago: University of Chicago, 1972), Research Series No. 30, Center for Health Administration Studies, pp. 12-3.

[20]*Ibid.*

Chapter 3

[1]Ernest Bergel, *Social Statification* (New York: McGraw-Hill, 1962), pp.331-3.

[2]Earl Lomon Koos, *The Sociology of the Patient* (New York: McGraw-Hill, 1959), pp. 97-8.

[3]M.W. Susser and W. Watson, *Sociology of Medicine* (London: Oxford University Press, 1971), pp. 130-8.

[4]*Ibid.*

[5]Raymond Wheeler, "Health and Human Resources," *New South* **9** (Fall 1971):2ff.

[6]George Tolbert, "Howard University Mississippi Health Project," *The New Physician* **19** (April 1970):319-24.

[7]Z.M. Stadt, "Socio-Economic Status and Dental Caries Experience of 3,911 Five-Year-Old Natives of Contra Costa County, California," *Journal of Public Health Dentistry* **27** (Winter 1967): 2-6.

[8]L. F. Szqejda, "Observed Differences of Total Caries Experience among White Children of Various Socio-Economic Groups," *Journal of Public Health Dentistry* **20** (Fall 1960):59-66.

[9]L. F. Szqejda, "Dental Caries Experience by Race and Socio-Economic Level After Eleven Years of Water Fluoridation in Charlotte, North Carolina," *Journal of Public Health Dentistry* **22** (Summer 1962):91-8.

[10]Earl Lomon Koos, *The Health of Regionville: What the People Thought and Did About It* (New York: Columbia University Press, 1954), pp. 118-25.

[11]*Ibid.*

[12]U.S. Department of Health, Education and Welfare, Public Health Service, *Decayed, Missing and Filled Teeth Among Youths 12-17 Years United States* (Washington, D.C.: U.S. Gov. Printing Office, 1974), p. 10.

[13]U.S. Department of Health, Education and Welfare, Public Health Service, *An Assessment of the Occlusion of the Teeth of Children 6-11 Years United States* (Washington, D.C.: U.S. Gov. Printing Office, 1973), p. 11.

[14]U.S. Department of Health, Education and Welfare, Public Health Service, *Periodontal Disease and Oral Hygiene Among Children United States* (Washington, D.C.: U.S. Gov. Printing Office, 1972), p. 6.

[15]U.S. Department of Health, Education, and Welfare, Public Health Service, *Edentulous Persons United States-1971* (Washington, D.C.: U.S. Gov. Printing Office 1974), p. 11.

[16]*Ibid.*, p. 4.

[17]John F. Newman and Odin W. Anderson, *Patterns of Dental Science Utilization in the United States: A Nationwide Survey* (Chicago: University of Chicago, 1972), Research Series No. 30, Center for Health Administration Studies, p. 23.

[18]*Ibid.*, p. 34.

[19]Peter F. Infants and George M. Owen, "Dental Caries and Levels of Treatment for School Children by Geographical Region, Socioeconomic Status, Race, and Size of Community," *Journal of Public Health Dentistry* **35** (Winter 1975):20-1.

[20]*Ibid.*

[21]L. A. Friedman et al., "Dental Survey of Houston Catholic Parochial School Children," *Texas Dental Journal* **11** (November 1971): 16-20.

[22]Jeannette F. Rayner, "Socioeconomic Status and Factors Influencing the Dental Health Practices of Mothers," *American Journal of Public Health* **60** (July 1970):1250-8.

[23]Donald L. Anderson, Gordon W. Thompson, and Frank Popvich, "Socioeconomic Status, Loss of Teeth, and Participation in a Dental Study," *Journal of Public Health Dentistry* **34** (Spring 1974):106-12.

[24]Clayton T. Shaw, "Class Characteristics of Supporters and Rejectors of Basic Health Measures," *Social Science and Medicine* **4** (November 1970):411-5.

[25]Mata K. Nikias et al., "Comparisons of Poverty and Non-Poverty Groups on Dental Status, Needs and Practices," *Journal of Public Health Dentistry* **35** (Fall 1975):256-8.

[26]David A. Nash and Sherwin R. Fishman, "Selected Dental Findings of a Rural Community in Appalachia," *Journal of Public Health Dentistry* **31** (Fall 1971):243-50.

[27]Richard A. Lewis, "Concern for Appalachia," *Journal of the American Dental Association* **82** (April 1971):684-7.

[28]William D. Lasser, "Missed Appointments: Most Are Not Ghetto-Related," *Dental Survey* **47** (March 1971):24.

[29]Donald W. Legler, Clyde W. Mayhall and Edwin L. Bradley, Jr., "Behavioral Characteristics of Disadvantaged Adult Patients," *Journal of Public Health Dentistry* **32** (Winter 1972):15-21.

[30]C. O. Enwonwu and J.C. Edozien, "Epidemiology of Periodontal

Disease in Western Nigerians in Relation to Socio-Economic Status," *Archives of Oral Biology* **15** (December 1970):1231-44.

[31] J. F. Beal and P.M. James, "Social Differences in the Dental Conditions and Dental Needs of 5-year-old Children in Four Areas of the West Midlands," *British Dental Journal* **129** (October 1970):313-8.

[32] Judith T. Shuval, "Social and Psychological Factors in Dental Health in Israel," *Milbank Memorial Fund Quarterly* **49** (July 1971):95-131.

[33] D. M. Roder, "The Dental Health and Habits of South Australian Children from Different Socioeconomic Environments," *Austrialian Dental Journal* **16** (February 1971):34-40.

[34] W. I. Vogan, "Dental Knowledge and Attitudes: An Investigation," *British Dental Journal* **128** (May 1970):481-6.

[35] Clifton O. Dummett, "Understanding the Underprivileged Patient," *Journal of the American Dental Association* **79** (December 1969):1363-7.

[36] *Ibid.*

Chapter 4

[1] Gordon Allport, *The Nature of Prejudice* (Cambridge, Mass.: Addison-Wesley, 1954), p. 108.

[2] *Ibid.*, p. 107

[3] Raymond W. Mack, ed., *Race, Class, and Power* (New York: American Book Co., 1963), p. 121.

[4] *Ibid.*, p. 118.

[5] *Ibid.*, p. 120

[6] *Ibid.*, p. 118.

[7] John Norman, ed., *Medicine in the Ghetto* (New York: Appleton-Century-Crofts, 1969), p. 33.

[8] *Social and Economic Status of the Black Population in the United States,* 1971; *Current Population Reports*, Series P-23, No. 42, U.S. Dept. of Commerce; *Handbook of Labor Statistics*, 1971, U.S. Dept. of Labor, p. 57; *Statistical Abstract of the United States*, 1972, p. 322.

[9] James A. Quinn, *Human Ecology* (Englewood Cliffs, N.J.: Prentice-Hall, 1950), p. 352.

[10] Melvin L. DeFleur, William V. D'Antonio, and Lois B. DeFleur, *Sociology: Human Society* (Glenview, Ill.: Scott, Foresman, 1976), pp. 243-44.

[11] *Ibid.*

[12] Charles F. Marden and Gladys Meyer, *Minorities in American Society* (New York: American Book Co., 1968), p. 23.

[13] U.S. Department of Health, Education, and Welfare, Public Health Service, *Minorities and Women in the Health Fields* (Washington, D.C.: U.S. Gov. Printing Office, 1975), p. 3.

[14] *Ibid.*, p. 50.

[15] *Ibid.*

[16] *Ibid.*, p. 51.

[17] Leon S. Robertson, John Kosa, Joel J. Alpert and Margaret C. Heagarty, "Race, Status, and Medical Care," *Phylon* **28** (Winter 1967):359.

[18] U.S. Department of Health, Education, and Welfare, Public Health

Service, *Examination and Health History Findings Among Children and Youths, 6-17 Years United States* (Washington, D.C.: U.S. Gov. Printing Office, 1973), p. 20.

[19]*Ibid.*

[20]*Ibid.*, pp. 25-6.

[21]U.S. Department of Health, Education, and Welfare, Public Health Service, Health Resources Administration, *Health, United States 1975* (Washington, D.C.: U.S. Gov. Printing Office, 1976), pp. 380-2.

[22]*Ibid.*, p. 454.

[23]*Ibid.*, 502-4.

[24]*Ibid.*, pp. 418-24.

[25]U.S. Department of Health, Education and Welfare, Public Health Service, Health Resources Administration, *Periodontal Disease Among Youth 12-17 Years United States* (Washington, D.C.: U.S. Gov. Printing Office, 1974), p. 5.

[26]U.S. Department of Health, Education and Welfare, Public Health Service, Health Resources Adminstration, *Oral Hygiene Among Youths 12-17 Years United States* (Washington, D.C.: U.S. Gov. Printing Office, 1975), p. 44.

[27]Richard F. Murphy, John T. Hughes, and George G. Dudney, "Dental Health Status of Students at the North Carolina Advancement School," *Journal of Public Health Dentistry* **30** (Fall 1970):234-8.

[28]R. A. Bagramian and A.L. Russell, "An Epidemiologic Study of Dental Caries in Race and Geographic Areas," *Journal of Dental Research* **50** (November-December 1971):1553-6.

[29]T. F. Varley and D. H. Goose, "Dental Caries in Children of Immigrants in Liverpool," *British Dental Journal* **130** (January 1971):27-9.

[30]M.E.J. Curzon and Jennifer A. Curzon, "Dental Caries in Eskimo Children of the Keewatin District in the Northwest Territories," *Journal of the Canadian Dental Association* **36** (September 1970):342-5.

[31]Anselm Langer, Julius Michman, and G. Librach, "Tooth Survival in a Multiracial Group of Aged in Israel," *Community Dentistry and Oral Epidemiology* **3** (May 1975):93-9.

[32]I. Yassin and T. Low, "Caries Prevalence in Different Racial Groups of School Children in West Malaysia," *Community Dentistry and Oral Epidemiology* **3** (August 1975):179-83.

[33]Kevin T. Avery, "The Oral Health Status of Migrant and Seasonal Farm Workers and Their Families," *Community Dentistry and Oral Epidemiology* **4** (January 1976):10-21.

[34]Martha B. Pointer and Eugena L. Mobley, "Dental Status and Needs in a Poverty-Population of North Nashville, Tennessee," *Journal of Public Health Dentistry* **29** (Fall 1969):4.

[35]Joseph Abramowitz, "Planning for the Indian Health Service," *Journal of Public Health Dentistry* **31** (Spring 1971):70-8.

Chapter 5

[1]Rodney M. Coe, *Sociology of Medicine* (New York: McGraw-Hill, 1970), p. 32.

[2]U.S. Department of Health, Education and Welfare, Public Health

Service, Health Resources Administration, *Health: United States 1975* (Washington, D.C.: U.S. Gov. Printing Office, 1975), p. 152.

[3] *Ibid.*, p. 176

[4] *Ibid.*, p. 178

[5] *Ibid.*, p. 188.

[6] *Ibid.*, p. 190

[7] *Ibid.*, p. 226.

[8] Earl L. Koos, *The Sociology of the Patient* (New York: McGraw-Hill, 1954), pp. 156-63.

[9] U.S. Department of Health, Education and Welfare, *Health: United States 1975*, p. 554.

[10] *Ibid.*, p. 556.

[11] *Ibid.*, p. 578.

[12] *Ibid.*, p. 582.

[13] *Ibid.*, 584.

[14] *Ibid.*, p. 592.

[15] *Ibid.*, p. 592-6.

[16] *Ibid.*, 200.

[17] *Ibid., pp. 202-4.*

[18] *Ibid.*, 206.

[19] U.S. Department of Health, Education and Welfare, Public Health Service, Health Resources Administration, *Selected Vital and Health Statistics in Poverty and Non-Poverty Areas of 19 Large Cities, United States, 1969-1971* (Washington, D.C.: U.S. Gov. Printing Office, 1975), p. 7.

[20] Koos, *Sociology of the Patient*, pp. 156-63.

[21] *Ibid.*

[22] U.S. Department of Health, Education and Welfare, *Health: United States 1975*, p. 224.

[23] *Ibid.*, pp. 234-6.

[24] U.S. Department of Health, Education and Welfare, *Selected Vital and Health Statistics for 19 Large Cities*, p. 10.

[25] U.S. Department of Health, Education, and Welfare, Public Health Service, Health Resources Administration, *Health Resources* (Washington, D.C.: U.S. Gov. Printing Office, 1976), p. 3.

[26] Koos, *The Sociology of the Patient*, pp. 156-63.

[27] R.J. Pryor, "Improving Dental Health Service to the Public," *Dental Student* **50** (January 1972):16.

[28] Bureau of Economic Research and Statistics, "1971 Survey of Dental Practice II: Income of Dentists by Location, Age, and Other Factors," *Journal of the American Dental Association* **84** (February 1972):397-402.

[29] Henry Wechsler, "Shortage in Dental Manpower: A Problem of Maldistribution," *Journal of Dental Education* **36** (January 1972):77-83.

[30] John M. Conchie, K.L. Scott and J.J. Philion, "A Simplified Method of Determining a Population's Need for Dental Treatment," *Journal of Public Health Dentistry* **31** (Spring 1971):84-95.

[31] R.W. Wilson, *The Sociology of Health: An Introduciton* (New York: Random House, 1970), p. 85.

[32] M. W. Susser and W. Watson, *Sociology in Medicine* (London: Oxford University Press, 1971), pp. 1-54.

[33] S. P. Ramjford, D.A. Kerr, and M. M. Ash, *World Workshop in Periodontics* (Ann Arbor: University of Michigan Press, 1969), p. 212.

[34] Susser and Watson, *Sociology in Medicine*, p. 27.

[35] K. Takagi et al., "Studies on the Future Demand for Dental Manpower in Japan II. Regional Distribution of Dentists," *Shikwa Gaku* **70** (April 1970):87-100.

[36] P. J. Chapman et al., "Dental Health of Pregnant Women I: Survey of Dental Knowledge, Attitudes and Practices in an Antenatal Clinic Population," *Medical Journal of Austrialia* **2** (November 27, 1971):1113-6.

[37]M. B. Edwards and J. D. Strahan, "Oral Hygiene Activity in a Selected Dental Population," *Dental Practitioner and Dental Record* **21** (May 1971):312-6.

[38]E. Kalliala-Hannukainen and H. Brusiin, "Oral Hygiene and Periodontal Conditions in a Group of Finnish Schoolchildren," *Suom Hammaslask Toim* **67** (1971):95-101.

[39]C. Olivieri Munroe, "The Oral Health of the Samaritan Community of Jordan," *Journal of Public Health Dentistry* **30** (Summer 1970):172-8.

[40]Mladen Kuftinec, "Oral Health in Guatemalan Rural Populations," *Journal of Dental Research* **50** (May-June 1971):559-64.

Chapter 6

[1]Anthony Downs, *Inside Bureaucracy* (Boston: Little, Brown, 1967), p. 24.

[2]Peter Blau and Marshall Meyer, *Bureaucracy in Modern Society* (New York: Random House, 1956), pp. 18-20.

[3]U.S. Department of Health, Education, and Welfare, Public Health Service, *Health Resources Statistics*, 1971 (Washington, D.C.: U.S. Gov. Printing Office, 1972), p. 77.

[4]Helen Constas, "Max Weber's Two Conceptions of Bureaucracy," *American Journal of Sociology* **63** (January 1958):400-9; as quoted in Francis E. Merrill, *Society and Culture* (Englewood Cliffs, N.J.: Prentice-Hall, 1963), pp. 351-2.

[5]Everett K. Wilson, *Sociology: Rules, Roles, and Relationships* (Homewood, Ill.: Dorsey Press, 1971), p. 357.

[6]Max Weber, *From Max Weber: Essays in Sociology*, trans. Hans Gerth and C. Wright Mills (New York: Oxford University Press, 1964).

[7]Alvin W. Gouldner, *Patterns of Industrial Bureaucracy* (New York: Free Press of Glencoe, 1954), pp. 181-228.

[8]*Ibid.*, p. 217

[9]U.S. Department of Health, Education, and Welfare, Public Health Service, Health Resources Administration, Bureau of Health Manpower, *A New Bureau: A Sharper Focus, Annual Report of Fiscal 1975 Activities* (Washington, D.C.: U.S. Gov. Printing Office, 1976), p. 2.

[10]*Health: United States 1978*, U.S. Dept. of Health, Education and Welfare, Public Health Service, DHEW Publication No. (PHS) 781232, December 1978.

[11]*Public Health Reports: Health Manpower,* **94** (January-February 1979), No. 1, p. 6.

[12]Herbert Freilich, "Written Communication," *Hospital Management* **109** (June 1970):31.

[13]Emily Mumford and James K. Skipper, *Sociology in Hospital Care* (New York: Harper & Row, 1967) pp. 127-8.

[14]American Dental Association, Council on Dental Education, Division of Educational Measurements, Annual Report 1972-73, *Dental*

Education Supplement, Minority Enrollment 1972, Auxiliary Programs (Chicago: The Association, 1973). American Dental Assoc. Council on Dental Education, Division of Educational Measurements, *Annual Report 1974-75, Dental Education Supplement 16, Auxiliary Programs Minority Report* (Chicago: The Association, 1975). Also previous edition.

[15]*Ibid.*

[16]*Ibid.*

[17]U.S. Department of Health, Education, and Welfare, Public Health Service, Health Resources Administration, Bureau of Health Manpower, *Minorities and Women in the Health Fields* (Washington, D.C.: U.S. Gov. Printing Office, 1975), pp. 48-9.

[18]Marcel Fredericks, Ralph Lobene and Paul Mundy, "A Model for Teaching Social Concepts to Dental Auxiliaries," *Journal of Dental Education* **35** (April 1971):232-5.

[19]Rodney M. Coe, *Sociology of Medicine* (New York: McGraw-Hill, 1970), pp. 268-9.

[20]*Ibid.*, p. 270.

[21]Mumford and Skipper, *Hospital Care*, p. 144.

[22]Stanley F. King, *Perceptions of Illness and Medical Practice* (New York: Russell Sage Foundation, 1962), pp. 307-48.

[23]Ronald G. Corwin, *A Sociology of Education* (New York: Appleton-Century-Crofts, 1965), p. 252.

[24]Robert K. Merton, *Social Theory and Social Structure* (Glencoe, Ill.: Free Press, 1949), pp. 151-60.

[25]*Ibid.*

[26]Coe, *Sociology in Medicine*, p. 288.

[27]Robert L. Dorfman, Leonard H. Kreit, and Dale W. Podshadley, "Dental Student Attitudes Toward Expanded Duties of Dental Assistants," *Journal of Dental Education* **35** (April 1971):220-4.

[28]Carl R. Koerner, "Dynamic Transition in Dentistry: Expanded Functions for Auxiliaries," *Journal of Public Health Dentistry* **31** (Spring 1971):123-40.

[29]Neil McKenzie and David O. Born, Dentists' Attitudes Toward Expanded Duties for Auxiliaries," *Journal of the American Dental Association* **86** (May 1973):1001-8.

[30]Leon Eisenbud, "The Form and Substance of a Hospital Dental Program," *Journal of the American Dental Association* **86** (May 1973):1039-44.

[31]Clifton O. Dummett, "Dentistry in Regional Medical Programs—Need for Greater Involvement," *American Journal of Public Health* **65** (May 1975):465-8.

[32]Robert A. Rothman, "Problems of Knowledge and Obsolescence Among Professionals: A Case Study in Dentistry," *Social Science Quarterly* **55** (December 1974):743-52.

[33]Richard Adelson, "The Role of the Hospital in Continuing Education," *Journal of Dental Education* **38** (September 1974):487-90.

[34]John Hedlin, "Education of Dental Auxiliaries," *Landstingens I* **58** (April 1971):27-34.

[35]T. Morstad, "Observation of the New Zealand Dental Nurse Plan," *Northwest Dentistry* **49** (September-October 1970):290-3.

Chapter 7

[1]Samuel W. Bloom, *The Doctor and His Patient* (New York: Russell Sage Foundation, 1963), p. 256.

[2]Lester J. Evans, *The Crisis in Medical Education* (Ann Arbor: University of Michigan Press, 1964), pp. 11-4.

[3]*Ibid.*

[4]James K. Skipper and Emily Mumford, *Sociology in Hospital Care* (New York: Harper & Row, 1967), pp. 127-8.

[5]*Ibid.*, p. 136.

[6]U.S. Department of Health, Education and Welfare, Public Health Service, Health Resources Administration, *Health: United States 1975* (Washington, D.C.: U.S. Gov. Printing Office, 1975), p. 103.

[7]U.S. Department of Health, Education and Welfare, Pubic Health Service, Health Resources Administration, *Health Manpower Issues: A Presentation at the White House* (Washington, D.C.: U.S. Gov. Printing Office, 1976), p. 7.

[8]*Ibid.*

[9]U.S. Department of Health, Education and Welfare, *Health: United States 1975*, p. 103.

[10]*Ibid.*, p. 106.

[11]U.S. Department of Health, Education and Welfare, Public Health Service, Health Resources Administration, *Group Dental Practice in the United States*, 1971 (Washington, D.C.: U.S. Gov. Printing Office, 1972), p. 447.

[12]*Ibid.*

[13]*Ibid.*

[14]*Ibid.*

[15]*Ibid.*, pp. 447-8.

[16]*Ibid.*

[17]Helen Gift and Karen A. Schaid, "Patterns of Dental Practice in the United States: Solo vs. Group Practice," *Journal of the American Dental Association* **91** (July 1975): 148-52.

[18]Richard E. Therrell, "The Plus Side of Group Practice for the Patient and Practitioner," *Dental Student* **50** (January 1972):26-7.

[19]Kerr Larence, "Group Practice Team," *Israeli Journal of Dental Medicine* **20** (October 1971):6-9.

[20]George Szasz, "Education for the Health Team," *Canadian Journal of Public Health* **61** (September-October 1970):386.

[21]Robert E. Pittman, "A New Kind of Group Practice," *Dental Student* **51** (March 1973):24.

[22]Irene R. Nantz, "Dental Hygiene's Changing Self-Concept," *Journal of the American Dental Hygiene Association* **45** (November-December 1971):373-7.

[23]Ralph R. Lobene, Marcel A. Fredericks and Paul Mundy, "Social Attitudes of Dental Hygiene Students: I," *Journal of the American Dental Hygiene Association* **45** (May-June 1971):164-8.

[24]Norman Gerrie, "A Proposed Functional Realignment System for Delivery of Oral Health Service," *Journal of the American College of Dentists* **39** (January 1972):29-41.

[25]Kathleen S. Kalal and Joanna Jenny, "Professional Aspirations, Job Satisfaction and Remuneration of Expanded Duty Dental Assistants," *The Dental Assistant* **42** (July 1973):14-8.

[26]L. V. Martens, L. H. Meskin and J. M. Proshek, "New Dental Care Concepts: Perceptions of Dentists and Dental Students," *American Journal of Public Health* **61** (November 1971):2188-94.

[27]S. Lotzkar, D. W. Johnson, and M. B. Thompson, "Experimental Program In Expanded Functions for Dental Assistants: Phase III Experiment with Dental Teams," *Journal of the American Dental Association* **82** (May 1971):1067-81.

[28]Gerald P. Hirsch et al., "Group Practice Revisited: How It's Working Out Now," *Dental Survey* **49** (November 1973):59-65.

[29]H. A. Zaki and R. E. Stallard, "The Role of the Dental Hygienist in Preventive Periodontics," *Journal of Periodontology* **42** (April 1971):233-6.

[30]Wilbur Hoff, "The Importance of Training for Effective Performance," *Public Health Reports* **85** (September 1970):760-5.

[31]Dixie C. Scoles, "Expanded Duties for the Dental Hygientist? Yes," *Journal of Dental Education* **35** (April 1971):209.

[32]Kenneth R. Rankin, "Debate of the 1970's: The Role of the Dental Auxiliary," *Journal of the Academy of General Dentistry* **19** (May 1971):9.

[33]Lawrence W. Loveland, "An Enlightened Conservative Look at Expanded Functions for Auxiliaries," *New York Journal of Dentistry* **41** (October 1971):280-2.

[34]Smiljko Slankamenac, "Psychological Aspects of Individual and Group Practice Administration," *Quintessence International* **5** (May 1974):65-71.

[35]Editorial, "Private Practice in the Seventies," *New Zealand Dental Journal* **67** (April 1971):75-8.

[36]G.P. Greenacres, "Dental Auxiliaries," *Journal of Canadian Dental Association* **9** (October 1972):591-3.

Chapter 8

[1]Ronald Warren, *The Community in America*, 2d ed. (Chicago: Rand McNally, 1972), p. 9.

[2]Ferdinand Tönnies, "On Gemeinschaft and Gesellschaft" trans. Charles P. Loomis in *Sociology: The Classic Statements*, ed. Marcello Truzzi (New York: Random House, 1971), pp. 145-54.

[3]U.S. Department of Health, Education and Welfare, Public Health Service, *Health Characteristics by Geographic Region, Large Metropolitan Areas, and Other Places of Residence United States – 1969-70* (Washington, D.C.: U.S. Gov. Printing Office, 1974), p. 13.

[4]Tönnies, "Gemeinschaft and Gesellschaft," p. 146.

[5]Ernest W. Burgess, "The Growth of the City," in *The City*, ed. Robert Park, Ernest Burgess and R.D. McKenzie (Chicago: University of Chicago Press, 1925).

[6]E. Franklin Frazier, "The Negro Family in Chicago," Ph.D. dissertation, University of Chicago, 1931.

[7]Joel J. Alpert, "Effective Use of Comprehensive Pediatric Care," *Journal of Diseases of Children* **116** (November 1968):529-33.

[8]U.S. Department of Health, Education and Welfare, Office of Public Affairs, "PHS Aims to Improve Health Care for Expanding Rural Population," HEW (October 1975):8.

[9]U.S. Department of Health, Education and Welfare, Public Health Service, Health Resources Administration, *Selected Vital and Health Statistics in Poverty and Nonpoverty Areas of 19 Large Cities United States, 1969-71* (Washington, D.C.: U.S. Gov. Printing Office, 1975), pp. 5-22.

[10]U.S. Department of Health, Education and Welfare, *Health United States 1975, a Chartbook* (Washington, D.C.: U.S. Gov. Printing Office, 1976), p. 46.

[11]*Ibid.*, pp. 36-41.

[12]*Ibid.*, p. 54.

[13]*Ibid.*, pp. 6-7.

[14]American Dental Association, "A Dental Program for the Community, State and Nation," in *Policies on Community Dental Health* (Chicago: American Dental Association, 1973), pp. 51-3.

[15]Clifton O. Dummett, "Dental Services in the Urban Community," *Journal of Dental Education* **35** (January 1971):12-6.

[16]Clifton O. Dummett, "Extramural Programs in Community Dentistry," *Journal of the American College of Dentists* **40** (October 1974):265.

[17]*Ibid.*, pp. 264-8.

[18]Thomas W. Wiggins and Donald E. Gibson, "Simulating Preventive Dentistry in the Community Perspective," *Journal of Dental Hygiene* **47** (May-June 1973):168-70.

[19]Wesley O. Young, "Changing Responsibilities of the Practitioner in Community Health," *Journal of Dentistry for Children* **39** (September-October 1972):45-9.

[20]Clifton O. Dummett, "Community Dentistry and Periodontology: A Reciprocal Affinity," *Journal of Periodontology* **44** (February 1973):106-10.

[21]Alice O. Ford, "The Community Dental Hygienist," *Dental Hygienist* **48** (November-December 1974):345-7.

[22]Nancy McCollum and Karen Jones, "St. Peter's: A Lesson in Community Involvement," *Journal of the American Dental Hygienists' Association* **45** (June 1971):172-5.

[23]H. Allred, M. H. Hobdell, and R. J. Elderton, "The Establishment of the Experimental Dental Care Project," *Journal of British Dentistry* **135** (September 1973):205-10.

[24]H. Colin Davis and J.D. Palmer, "The Dental Student in the Community," *British Dental Journal* **137** (September 1974):191-3.

[25]D. Jackson, "Measuring Restorative Dental Care in Communities," *British Dental Journal* **134** (May 1973):385-8.

[26]Herschel S. Horowitz, "A Review of Systemic and Topical Fluorides for the Prevention of Dental Caries," *Community Dentistry and Oral Epidemiology* **1** (1973):104-14.

[27]D. Jackson J.J. Murray, and C.G. Fairpo, "Life-long Benefits of Fluoride in Drinking Water," *British Dental Journal* **134** (May 1973):419-22.

[28]Sidney Epstein, "Responsibility of the Hospital to Multiphasic Community Dental Care," *Journal of California Dental Association* **2** (February 1974):44-9.

[29]*Ibid.*

[30]Editorial, "Group," *Dental Student* **52** (January 1974):30-4.

[31]Brian A. Burt and G.L. Slack, "Dental Data Requirements in the Area Health Authorities," *British Dental Journal* **135** (October 1973):361-4.

[32]Editorial, "The Area Dental Officer," *British Dental Journal* **136** (March 1974):177-78.

Chapter 9

[1]U.S. Department of Health, Education and Welfare, Public Health Service, *Health United States 1975* (Washington, D.C.: U.S. Gov. Printing Office, 1976), p. 542.

[2]"A Profile of Older Americans," *U.S. News and World Report* **80** (February 23, 1976):71.

[3]Ernest W. Burgess, "The Growth of a City," in *The City*, ed. by Robert E. Park, Ernest W. Burgess, and Roderick D. McKenzie (Chicago: University of Chicago Press, 1925), pp. 47-62.

[4]Ira Robbins, *Housing the Elderly*, White House Conference on Aging (Washington, D.C.: U.S. Gov. Printing Office, 1971), p. 6.

[5]Donald O. Cowgill, "The Demography of Aging," in *The Daily Needs and Interests of Older People*, ed. by Adeline M. Hoffman (Springfield, Ill.: Charles C. Thomas, 1970), p. 65.

[6]*Ibid.*, pp. 56-7.

[7]*Ibid.*

[8]"A Profile of Older Americans," p. 71.

[9]*Ibid.*

[10]David Moberg, *Spiritual Well-Being,* White House Conference on Aging (Washington, D.C.: U.S. Gov. Printing Office, 1971), p. 14.

[11]Minnie Field, *Aging with Honor and Dignity* (Springfield, Ill. Charles C. Thomas, 1968), p. 13.

[12]Gordon Streib, *Retirement Roles and Activities*, White House Conference on Aging (Washington, D.C.: U.S. Gov. Printing Office, 1971), p. 1.

[13]Elaine M. Brody and Stanley J. Brody, "Decade of Decision for the Elderly," *Social Work* **19** (September 1974):548.

[14]George L. Maddox, "Persistence of Life Style Among the Elderly: A Longitudinal Study of Patterns of Social Activity in Relation to Life Satisfaction," in Bernice L. Neugarten, ed., *Middle Age and Aging* (Chicago: University of Chicago Press, 1968), pp. 181-5.

[15]Elaine Cumming and William H. Henry, *Growing Old: The Process of Disengagement* (New York: Basic Books, 1961).

[16]Ethel Shanas, *The Health of Older People* (Cambridge, Mass.: Harvard University Press, 1962), p. 53.

[17]U.S. Department of Health, Education and Welfare, Public Health Service, *Health United States, 1975*, p. 550.

[18]Field, *Aging with Honor and Dignity*, p. 12.

[19]*Health United States, 1975*, p. 552.

[20]*Ibid.*

[21]*Ibid.*, p. 562.

[22]*Ibid.*, p. 594.

[23]Neil Solomon, Nathan Shook and Patricia Aughenbaugh, "The Biology of Aging," in Hoffman, ed., *The Daily Needs and Interests of Older People*, p. 196.

[24]*Ibid.*, p. 200.

[25]*Ibid.*, p. 202.

[26]Austin Chinn, Edward Colby, and Edith Robins, *Physical and Mental Health*, White House Conference on Aging (Washington, D.C.: U.S. Gov. Printing Office, 1971), p. 3.

[27]*Ibid.*, p. 18.

[28]Eugene Confrey and Marcus Goldstein, "The Health Status of Aging People," in *Handbook of Social Gerontology*, ed. Clark Tibbits (Chicago: University of Chicago Press, 1960), p. 176.

[29]Some of the problems of medical care are graphically presented in Bernard Isaacs, Maureen Livingstone, and Yvonne Neville, *Survival of the Unfittest: A Study of Geriatric Patients in Glasgow* (London: Routledge and Kegan Paul, 1972).

[30]Field, *Aging with Honor*, p. 14.

[31]*Ibid.*, p. 49.

[32]Chinn, Colby and Robins, *Physical and Mental Health*, pp. 52-4.

[33]Robert E. Vestal, "Geriatric Pharmacology: Current Status and Future Prospects," paper presented in the Science Writers' Seminar on Aging Research, at the Gerontology Research Center, NIA, NIH, Baltimore, October 1, 1976.

[34]U.S. Department of Health, Education and Welfare, Public Health Service, *National Institute on Aging* (Washington, D.C.: U.S. Gov. Printing Office, 1976).

[35]*Ibid.*

[36]*Ibid.*

[37]R. H. Gordon, "Meeting Dental Health Needs of the Aged," *American Journal of Public Health* **62** (March 1972):385-8.

[38]Myron Allukian, Norma De Jong, and James M. Dunning, "Caring for Nursing Home Patients—Learning Experience for Dental Students," *Journal of Dental Education* **36** (September 1972):45-8.

[39]Arthur Elfenbaum, "Dentures Are Not for All the Edentulous," *Dental Digest* **78** (January 1972):24-7.

[40]J. D. Manson, "The Elderly Dental Cripple," *Proceedings of the Royal Society of Medicine* **66** (June 1973): 597-8.

[41]Mikael Grabowski and Ulrik Bertram, "Oral Health Status and Need of Dental Treatment in the Elderly Danish Population," *Community Dentistry and Oral Epidemiology* **3** (May 1975):108-14.

[42]Robert Cutler, "The Fifth Commandment," *British Dental Journal* **136** (April 1974):341-2.

[43]A. S. T. Franks and G. B. Winter, "Management of the Handicapped and Chronic Sick Patient in Dental Practice," *British Dental Journal* **134** (February 1974):145-50.

[44]Ronald L. Ettinger, "An Evaluation of the Attitudes of a Group of Elderly Edentulous Patients to Dentists, Dentures and Dentistry," *The Dental Practitioner and Dental Record* **22** (November 1971):85-91.

[45]J. S. Gerrish, A. Yardley, G. D. Stafford, and J. F. Bates, "A Dental Survey of People Living in Residential Homes for the Elderly in Cardiff," *Dental Practitioner and Dental Record* **22** (July 1972):433-5.

[46]G. M. Ritchie, "A Report of Dental Findings in a Survey of Geriatric Patients," *Journal of Dentistry* **1** (February 1973):106-12.

[47]M. R. Heath, "Dietary Selection by Elderly Persons, Related Dental State," *British Dental Journal* **132** (February 1972):145-8.

[48]Maury Massler, "Geriatric Care in Israel," *Journal of the American Society of Geriatric Dentistry* **6** (April 1971):3.

Chapter 10

[1]David C. McClelland, *The Achieving Society* (Princeton, N.J.: Van Nostrand Press, 1961).

[2]Everett E. Hagen, *On the Theory of Social Change* (London: Tavistock, 1964).

[3]U.S. Department of Health, Education and Welfare, Public Health Service, *Hospital Discharges and Length of Stay: Short-Stay Hospitals United States—1972* (Washington, D.C.: U.S. Gov. Printing Office 1976), p. 17.

[4]U.S. Department of Health, Education and Welfare, Public Health Service, *Inpatient Health Facilities as Reported from the 1973 MFI Survey* (Washington, D.C.: U.S. Gov. Printing Office, 1976), p. 3.

[5]*Ibid.*

[6]*Ibid.*, p. 12.

[7]*Ibid.*, p. 13.

[8]*Ibid.*, p. 15.

[9]*Ibid.*, p. 14.

[10]Wesley O. Young, "Changing Responsibilities of the Practitioner in Community Health," *Journal of Dentistry for Children* **39** (September-October 1972):379-84.

[11]Hubert J. Bell, Presidential Address, American Assocation of Orthodontists at the Dallas Meeting, May 16, 1973, *American Journal of Orthodontics* **64** (August 1973):197-8.

[12]Kenneth V. Randolph, "The Dental Examiner and Our Changing Society," *The Journal of the American College of Dentists* **41** (April 1974):92-102.

[13]H. Hillenbrand, "Changing Social Attitudes to Dental Health," *Israeli Journal of Dental Medicine* **20** (October 1971):3-5.

[14]Jean M. Poupard, "The Future of Dental Auxiliaries in the Changing World Scene," *Journal of the American Dental Hygienists' Association* **45** (January-February 1971):34-43.

[15]Richard B. Weinber, "Future Dental Shock," *Dental Student* **50** (December 1971):20-2.

[16]Norman H. Rickles, "Dental Futures: Calculated Risks," *The Journal of the Oregon Dental Associates* **41** (February 1972):6-8.

[17]Editorial: "The Future of Dentistry," *Dental Cosmos* **14** (November 18, 1972):610.

[18]Ralph R. Lobene, "Clinicians' View of Future Dental Practitioners," *Journal of Dental Education* **36** (August 1972):41-4.

[19]Ralph R. Lobene et al., "The Forsyth Experiment in Training of Advanced Skills Hygienists," *Journal of Dental Education* **38** (August 1972):369-79.

Bibliography

Anderson, R., Greeley, R., Kravits, J., and O. Anderson. 1972. *Health Service Use. National Trends and Variations 1953-1971.* Contract No. HSM-73-3004.

Austin, G., Maher, M., and C. Lomonaco. 1973. Women in Dentistry and Medicine: Attitudinal Study of Educational Experience. *Journal of Dental Education* **38**:11.

Barber, Bernard, 1973. *Research on Human Subjects.* New York: Russell Sage Foundation.

Barnes, Donna P. 1976. Social Perspective on Community Dental Health. *Dental Hygiene* **50**:457-62.

Beecher, Henry K. 1970. *Research and the Individual.* Boston: Little, Brown.

Bell, D. 1972. Prosthodontic Failures Related to Improper Patient Education and Lack of Patient Acceptance. *Dental Clinic North America* **16**:109

Bissell, Donald G. 1975. Student Participation in Community Dental Health Programs: The Experience at SUNY at Buffalo. *Journal of Dental Education* **39**:517-21.

Bluitt, Juliann. 1974. Women's Place in Dentistry Is Changing. *Dental Student* **52**:26-8.

________. 1976. The Change of the Seventies Regarding Dental Auxiliaries. *Journal of Dental Education* **40**:200-2.

Bureau of Economic Research and Statistics. 1974. *Distribution of Dentists in the United States by State, Region, District, and County.* Chicago: American Dental Association.

________. 1973. *Distribution of Orthodontists by State, City, and Federal Dental Service 1973.* Chicago: American Dental Association.

________. 1973. Growth in Population and Number of Dentists to 1985. *Journal of the American Dental Association* **87**:901.

________. 1973. *The 1971 Survey of Dental Practice.* Chicago: American Dental Association.

Cain, Ella. 1974. Expanded Duty Assistants. *The Dental Assistant* **43**:22-7.

Callahan, D. 1973. The WHO Definition of Health. *The Hastings Center Studies* **1**:77-8.

Campbell, J. 1970. Women Dentists – An Untapped Resource. *Journal of the American College of Dentists* **37**:265.

Chung, C., Runck, D., Niswander, J., Bilben, S., and M. Dan. 1970. Genetic and Epidemiological Studies of Oral Characteristics in Hawaii's Schoolchildren: I. Caries and Periodontal Disease. *Journal of Dental Research* **49**:1374.

Cochrane, A.L. 1972. *Effectiveness and Efficiency: Random Reflections on Health Services*. London: Nuffield Provincial Hospitals Trust.

Cohen L., and H. Horowitz. 1970. Occlusal Relations in Children Born and Reared in an Optimally Fluoridated Community. III. Sociophysical Findings. *Angle Orthodontist* **40**:159.

________, and J. Jago. 1976. Toward the Formulation of Sociodental Indicators. *International Journal of Health Services* **6**:681.

Cooper, Michael. 1975. *Rationing Health Care*. New York: John Wiley (Halsted Press).

Croog, S., Lipson, A., and S. Levine. 1972. Help Patterns in Severe Illness: The Roles of Kin Network, Non-Family Resources, and Institutions. *Journal of Marriage and the Family* **34**:32-41.

Darby, Michele, and Susan Schwartz. 1977. Status of Dental Auxiliaries: An Issue of Gender? *The Dental Hygienist* 51:271-6.

Davis, K. 1975. *National Health Insurance: Benefits, Costs, and Consequences*. Washington, D.C.: Brookings Institute.

Davis, M. 1971. Variation in Patients' Compliance with Doctor's Orders: Medical Practice and Doctor-Patient Interaction. *Psychiatry in Medicine* **2**:31.

DeGeyndt, W. 1973. Health Behavior and Health Needs of Urban Indians in Minneapolis. *Health Services Report* **88**:360.

Denenberg, H. 1973. *Shopper's Guide to Surgery*. Harrisburg: State of Pennsylvania.

Douglass, Chester W., and Katherine O. Cole. 1979. The Supply of Dental Manpower in the United States. *Journal of Dental Education* **43**:287-301.

Dubos, Rene. 1972. *A God Within*. New York: Scribner's.

Dummett, Clifton O. 1970. The Vanishing Minority Dentist. *Journal of the American College of Dentists* **37**:256-63.

________. 1971. Dental Services in the Urban Community. *Journal of Dental Education* **35**:12-6.

________. 1973. Consumer-Provider Conflict in Health Service Recommendations. *Health Service Reports* **88**:795.

________. 1974. Extramural Programs in Community Dentistry. *Journal of the American College of Dentists* **40**:264-8.

________. 1977. Health Care and Community Dentistry. *Journal of Indiana Dental Association* **56**:22-6.

Dunning, James. 1970. Ecology and the Family Dentist. *New York Journal of Dentistry* **40**:195-200.

Durban, E. 1973. What's the Hang-Up? *Dental Economics* **63**:42.

Fewell, R. D. 1977. The Value of Increased Utilization of Auxiliary Personnel in Orthodontics. M.S. thesis, University of Tennessee, Memphis.

Fletcher, Joseph. 1974. *The Ethics of Genetic Control: Ending Reproductive Roulette*. Garden City, N.Y.: Anchor Press/Doubleday.

Fox, R. C. 1977. The Medicalization and Demedicalization of American Society. *Daedalus* **106**:9-22.

Fredericks, M. A., Lobene, R.R., and P. Mundy. 1971. A Model for Teaching Social Concepts to Dental Auxiliaries. *Journal of Dental Education* **35**:232-5.

________, ________, ________. 1972. Teaching Dental Auxiliaries the Interactional Aspects of Social Concepts. *Journal of Dental Education* **36**:37-40.

________, Mundy, P., and J. Lennon. 1972. The Student-Dentist and the Poor: A Study of Expressed Willingness to Serve the Indigent Patient. *Journal of the American College of Dentists* **39**:84-90.

________, ________, and R.R. Lobene. 1972. The Relationship Between Social Class, Stress Anxiety Responses, Achievement and Professional Attitudes of Dental Hygiene Students. *Journal of the American Dental Hygienists Association* **46**:113-7.

________, ________, and L. Blanchet. 1973. The Relationship Between Social Class, Academic Achievement and National Board Scores in a Dental School. *Journal of the American College of Dentists* **40**:174-81.

________, ________, ________. 1973. Dental Auxiliaries and the Poor: Study of Expressed Willingness to Serve. *Dental Student* **51**:41-3.

________, and P. Mundy. 1973. *Sociology of Health Care,* Chicago: Loyola University.

________, ________, and L. Blanchet. 1975. Dental Students: Social Class and National Board Scores. *Ohio Dental Journal* **49**:32-4.

________, Lobene, R.R., and P. Mundy. 1975. The Teaching of Demographic Components in the Behavioral Sciences to Dental Hygienists. *Dental Hygiene* **49**:352-5.

________, and P. Mundy. 1976. *The Making of a Physician* (Ten Year Longitudinal Study). Chicago: Loyola University Press.

________, Lobene, R.R., and P. Mundy. 1976. A Model for Teaching the Concepts of Bureaucracy. *Educational Directions* **1**:14-9.

________, Mundy, P., and R. Lobene. 1977. A Model for Teaching the Interactional Aspects of Social Concepts in Dental Health Care. *Educational Directions* **2**:7-13.

________, ________, ________. 1978. A Model for Teaching the Components of Society-Culture-Personality (SCP) in Dental Care. *Educational Directions* **3**:12-9.

Frome, David H. 1973. Health Maintenance Organization: A Future for Dentistry? *Georgetown Dental Journal* **38**:11-4.

Fuchs, Victor R. 1974. *Who Shall Live? Health, Economics, and Social Choice*. New York: Basic Books.

________. 1976. From Bismarck to Woodcock: "The 'Irrational' Pursuit of National Health Insurance. Center for Economic Analysis of Human Behavior and Social Institutions, Working Paper No. 120. National Bureau of Economic Research.

Fusillo, A., and A.S. Metz. 1971. Social Science Research on the Dental Student. In Richards, N.D., and L. Cohen, eds., *Social Sciences and Dentistry: A Critical Bibliography*. The Hague: Fédération Dentaire Internationale.

Galiher, Claudia B. 1975. Consumer Acceptance of HMO's. *Public Health Reports* **90**:106-12.

Garland, M. 1976. Politics, Legislation, and Natural Death. *The Hastings Center Report* **6**:5-6.

Gift, Helen C. 1978. Social and Psychological Barriers to Dental Care: Consideration of the Near-Poverty Income Individual. *Journal of the American College of Dentists* **45**:170-83.

Gilman, C.W. 1972. The Interface of Dental Assisting and Dentistry 1887-1987. *The Dental Assistant* **41**:11-2.

Glaser, W.A. 1970. *Social Settings and Medical Organization*. New York: Atherton.

Glazier, W.H. 1973. The Task of Medicine. *Scientific American* **228**:13-7.

Glazzard, Margaret, and M. Williams. 1977. The "Team Approach" to Patient Care in a Major Health Center. *Dental Survey,* **53**:10, 12, 14, 16, 20.

Gove, W.R. 1973. Sex, Marital Status, and Mortality. *American Journal of Sociology* **79**:45-67.

Haber, Lawrence, and Richard Smith. 1971. Disability and Deviance: Normative Adaptation of Role Behavior. *American Sociological Review* **36**:87-97.

Handler, Philip. 1970. *Biology and the Future of Man*. New York: Oxford University Press.

Henry, J. 1970. Bridging the Gap. *Journal of the American College of Dentists* **37**:249.

Henry, Joseph L., and Jeanne C. Sinkford. 1973. Recruitment of Minorities for the Health Professions. *Health Services Reports* **88**:113-6.

Hetherington, Robert. 1975. *Health Insurance Plans: Promise and Performance*. New York: Wiley-Interscience.

Hilgenrath, S. 1970. Social and Psychological Factors Related to Malocclusion and the Seeking of Orthodontic Treatment. M.S. thesis, Harvard University.

Hirsch, B., Levin, B., and N. Tiber. 1973. Effects of Dentist

Authoritarianism on Patient Evaluation of Dentures. *Journal of Prosthetic Dentistry* **30**:745.

Ho, S. 1976. New York State Registered Dental Hygienists: A Survey of Their Employment Status, Job Responsibilities, Career Satisfaction and Expectations. M.S. Thesis, State University of New York at Stony Brook.

House, Donald R. 1978. Barriers to Access to Dental Care: An Economic Examination. *Journal of the American College of Dentists* **45**:160-87.

Howard, Jan, and Anselm Strauss, eds. 1975. *Humanizing Health Care.* New York: Wiley-Interscience.

Huntington, J. 1973. Distant Early Warning System for Your Practice. *Dental Management* **13**:52.

Hyman, M.D. 1972. Social Isolation and Performance in Rehabilitation. *Journal of Chronic Disease* **25**:85-97.

Illich, I. 1976. *Medical Nemesis: The Expropriation of Health.* New York: Pantheon.

Jacobs, R.M., ed. 1976. *A Flexible Design for Health Professions Education: Medicine, Dentistry, Pharmacy, Nursing, Allied Health.* New York: Wiley.

Jenny, J. 1975. A Social Perspective on Need and Demand for Orthodontic Treatment. *International Dental Journal* **25**:248.

Johnson, D., and F. Holz. 1975. Legal Provisions on Expanded Functions for Dental Hygienists and Assistants; summarized by state 1973. Bethesda, Md., *Division of Dentistry* **97.**

________, Bissell, D., O'Shea, R., and A. Trithart. 1970. Dental Student Orientation Program to Community Health Problems. *Journal of Dental Education* **35**:156-64.

Jones, R. 1972. Dentists' Views on Reimbursement Arrangements Under Prepayment and Insurance Plans. *Journal of the American Dental Association* **84**:125.

Katz, E., and B. Danet. 1973. Petitions and Persuasive Appeals: A Study c Official-Client Relations. In Katz, E., and Danet, B., eds., *Bureaucracy and the Public.* New York: Basic Books.

Kennedy, E. 1972. *In Critical Condition.* New York: Simon & Schuster.

Klarman, E. 1977. The Financing of Health Care. *Daedalus* **106**:215-34.

Kleinknecht, R., Klepac, R., and L. Alexander. 1973. Origins and Characteristics of Fear of Dentistry. *Journal of the American Dental Association* **86**:842.

Korsch, B., and V. Negrete. 1972. Doctor-Patient Communication. *Scientific American* **230**:66.

Krause, E. 1977. *Power and Illness: The Political Sociology of Health and Medical Care.* New York: Elsevier.

Ladimer, I., ed. 1970. New Dimensions in Legal and Ethical Concepts for Human Research. *Annals of the New York Academy of Sciences* **169**:584-93.

Landy, D., ed. 1977. *Culture, Disease and Healing: Studies in Medical Anthropology*. New York: Macmillan.

Langlie, J. 1977. Social Networks, Health Beliefs, and Preventive Health Behavior. *Journal of Health and Social Behavior* **18**:244-60.

Leslie, G., and D. Leverett. 1976. Variables Affecting Attitudes of Dentists Toward the Use of Expanded Function Auxiliaries. *Journal of Dental Education* **40**:79-88.

Linn, E. 1970. Professional Activities of Women Dentists. *Journal of American Dental Association* **81**:1383-7.

________. 1972. Women Dentists: Some Circumstances about Their Choice of a Career. *Journal of Canadian Dental Association* **10**:364-9.

________. 1972. Black Dentists: Some Circumstances about Their Occupational Choice. *Journal of Dental Education* **36**:25-30.

Lobene, Ralph. 1966. The Evaluation of Oral Hygiene in Preventive Dentistry. *Journal of Massachusetts Dental Society* **15**:158-64.

________, Fredericks, M., and P. Mundy. 1970. Social Attitudes of Students of Dental Assisting. *The Dental Assistant* **39**:16-9.

________, ________, ________. 1970. Social Attitudes of Students of Dental Assisting—Part II, Professional Concerns. *The Dental Assistant* **39**:16-9.

________, ________, ________. 1970. Social Attitudes of Students of Dental Assisting—Part III, Service to the Economically Disadvantaged. *The Dental Assistant* **39**:17-20.

________. 1971. How to Motivate Patients Toward Effective and Permanent Oral Health. *Parodontologie* **25**:58-9.

________, Fredericks, M., and P. Mundy. 1971. Analysis of Board Certification and Personality Characteristics of Dental Assisting Students. *The Dental Assistant* **40**:17-21.

________. 1972. What Is the Future Role of Auxiliaries in Periodontics? *Periodontics Abstract* **20**:157.

Logan, R. F. L. 1971. National Health Planning—An Appraisal of the State of the Art. *International Journal of Health Services* **1**:6-17.

Maddich, Jan. 1972. The Community Dentist. *Community Health* **4**:125-7.

Masters, Leslie, Loupe, M., Modun, L., and Anthony Diangelis. 1975. Patient Views on Team Dentistry and Expanded Duties. *The Dental Hygienist* **49**:305-10.

McKinlay, J. B. 1972. Some Approaches and Problems in the Study of the Use of Services—An Overview. *Journal of Health and Social Behavior* **13**:115-52.

McLean, L. Deckle. 1973. Master Plan Supports Team Approach. *Journal of the New Jersey Dental Association* **44**:8-10.

Meskin, H. 1977. Too Many Dentists? If So, What Then? *Journal of Dental Education* **44**:601-5.

Miller, S. 1970. *Prescriptions for Leadership: Training for the Medical Elite.* Chicago: Aldine.

Milgrom, Peter, Nash, J., and Sheldon Rohn. 1974. Identifying Leadership Careers in the Dental Profession. *Journal of Dental Education* **38**:140-6.

Mulvihill, James E. 1976. Barriers to Identification and Motivation of Minority Group Members for Dentistry. *Journal of Dental Education* **40**:142-6.

Nelsen, Robert J. 1976. The Effect of the Third-Party Payment System on the Profession. *Journal of the American College of Dentists* **43**:103-11.

Newhouse, Joseph P., Phelps, C.E., and William B. Schwartz. 1974. Policy Options and the Impact of National Health Insurance. *Journal of the California Dental Association* **2**:50-64.

Newman, J., and O. Anderson. 1972. *Patterns of Dental Service Utilization in the United States: A Nationwide Social Survey.* Center for Health Administration Studies. Chicago: University of Chicago.

Nikias, Mata K., Fink, R., and Sam Shapiro. 1975. Comparisons of Poverty and Nonpoverty Groups on Dental Status, Needs and Practices. *Journal of Public Health Dentistry* **35**:237-59.

Obuhoff, Oleg N. 1976. Growing Up to the Maximum Use of Auxiliaries. *Journal of the Massachusetts Dental Society* **25**:80-6.

O'Daniel, Delores. 1973. Dental Auxiliary Identity Crises. *The Dental* Assistant **42**:19-22.

Parsons, Talcott. 1975. The Sick Role and the Role of the Physician Reconsidered. *Health and Society* **53**:257-78.

Pearson, David A., and Barry Goldberg. 1975. Elements of Progressive Patient Care in the Yale Health Plan HMO. *Public Health Reports* **90**:119-25.

Perlus, Jon D. 1972. Socioeconomic Status and the Utilization of Dental Services. *McGill Dental Review* **34**:9-11.

Peterson, S., ed. 1977. *Comprehensive Review of Dental Hygienists.* St. Louis: Mosby.

________, ed. 1977. *The Dentist and the Assistant.* St. Louis: Mosby.

Phillips, Lloyd J. 1974. The Wonderful World of Prepayment. *Ohio Dental Journal* **48**:12-5.

Powell, W.O. 1975. Demonstrating the Dentist-Dental Hygienist Team. Final report: Dental Therapist Training Project, College of Dentistry, Howard University. Prepared for National Center for Health Services Research, Washington, D.C.

Public Awareness Shows Growing Understanding and Support (Editorial). 1975. *Texas Dental Journal* **93**:24-7.

Ramsey, Paul. 1970. *The Patient as a Person*. New Haven, Conn.: Yale University Press.

Reports of Councils and Bureaus. 1974. Making Dental Care Available to the People in Between—Council on Dental Health. *Journal of the American Dental Association* **89**:906-8.

Rhodes Directory of Black Dentistry. 1973. Distribution of Black Dentists and Black Population in 1970-1971 by Regions and States and Population per Black Dentist in the U.S., pp. 44-5.

Richardson, R.E., and R.E. Barton. 1978. *The Dental Assistant*. New York: McGraw-Hill.

Richardson, S. 1970. Age and Sex Differences in Values Toward Physical Handicaps. *Journal of Health and Social Behavior* **11**:207.

Robinson, Emerson. 1974. Dental Hygiene Students in Community Dentistry: An Extramural Program at the University of Michigan. *Journal of the Michigan Dental Association* **56**:74-6.

Roghman, Klaus J., and Elbert A. Powell. 1974. Impact of Medicaid and an OEO Health Center on Use of Dental Services in an Urban Area. *Public Health Reports* **89**:325-9.

Schoen, William P., and James Brophy. 1976. All about Women Dentists. *Illinois Dental Journal* **45**:268-72.

Schwartz, B. 1974. Waiting, Exchange and Power: The Distribution of Time in Social Systems. *American Journal of Sociology* **79**:841.

Scott, R., and A. Howard. 1970. Models of Stress. In Levine, S., and N.A. Scotch, eds., *Social Stress*. Chicago: Aldine.

Selig, Andrew L. 1976. Delivery of Services—A Conceptual Framework for Evaluating Human Service Delivery Systems. *American Journal of Orthopsychiatry* **46**:140-53.

Siegler, M. and H. Osmond. 1973. The Sick Role Revisited. *The Hastings Center Studies* **1**:41-58.

Sinkford, Jeanne C. 1976. Current Status and Future Trends in Training Dental Practitioners and Dental Auxiliaries to Meet the Needs of the Black Community. *Journal of the National Medical Association* **68**:60-3.

Soble, Rosalynde, and Harris Chaiklin. 1973. Helping Inner-City Families Obtain Preventive Dentistry for Their Preschool Children. *Child Welfare* **52**:602-10.

Somers, Anne R. 1978. The High Cost of Health Care for the Elderly: Diagnosis, Prognosis, and Some Suggestions for Therapy. *Journal of Health Politics, Policy and Law* **3**:163-80.

Stauffer, E. 1972. Hospitals and Health Centers in Community Health: U.S.C. Health Services Center Program. *National Dental Association Quarterly* **30**:28-31.

Stevens, R. 1971. What Dental Boards Are Doing about Auxiliaries. *Journal of Public Health Dentistry* **31**:109-16.

Thompson, R., Jr. 1970. Considerations Involving the Shortage of Black Dentists. *Journal of Dental Education* **34**:399-401.

Torres, H. 1973. The Task Before Us—Part II. *The Dental Assistant* **42**:17-8.

________. 1973. A Look at Where We Have Been and Where We Are in Dental Assisting—Part 1. *The Dental Assistant* **36**:19-23.

Tryon, Aines F. 1974. Factors Influencing Variations in Distribution of Dental Manpower in an Urban Area. *Public Health Reports* **89**:320-4.

U.S. Division of Dentistry. Should You Add an Expanded Function Dental Auxiliary to Your Staff? Bethesda, Md.: Health Manpower References.

Verbrugge, L. 1975. Morbidity and Mortality in the United States. Unpublished paper, Department of Social Relations and Center for Metropolitan Planning and Research, Johns Hopkins University, Baltimore.

Waldman, H. 1972. Usual and Customary: Philosophy and Fees. *Annals of Dentistry* **31**:36.

________. 1977. Departments of Community Dentistry—Are They a Threat to the Dental Profession? *Journal of American College of Dentists* **44**:80-109.

Webb, H. Jr. 1974. An Enigma for Dentistry—HMO. *Ohio Dental Journal* **48**:20-30.

Welch, Susan, Comer, J., and M. Steinman. 1973. Some Social and Attitudinal Correlates of Health Care Among Mexican Americans. *Journal of Health and Social Behavior* **14**:205-13.

Whiteman, James. 1975. The National Health Planning and Resources Development Act. *Journal of Missouri Dental Association* **55**:10-5.

Widdison, Harold, and J. Skipper, Jr. 1970. The Mormon Dental Student Profile. *Journal of Dental Education* **34**:62-70.

Wildavsky, A. 1977. Doing Better and Feeling Worse: The Political Pathology of Health Policy. *Daedalus* **106**:105-23.

Wilson, Robert, and Samuel Bloom. 1972. Patient-Practitioner Relationship. In Freeman H., Levine, S., and L.G. Reeder, eds., *Handbook of Medical Sociology*. Englewood Cliffs, N.J.: Prentice-Hall.

Wirthlin, Robert. 1973. Periodontics and National Health Legislation. *Periodontal Abstracts* **21**:13-6.

Woodall, I.R. 1977. *Leadership, Management, and Role Delineation: Issues for the Dental Team*. St. Louis: C.V. Mosby.

Workshop on Dental Auxiliary Expanded Functions: Proceedings. 1976. March 31, April 1-2, Chicago. American Dental Association, Council on Dental Education.

Workshop on Minority Dental Student Recruitment, Retention, and Education: Proceedings. 1975. April 24-26, Kansas City, Mo.

Workshop Proceedings on Current and Future Dental Roles in Primary Care. October 9-10, 1975, Bethesda, Md., and April 8-9, 1976,

Washington, D.C. Ed. by Meskin, Lawrence H., Loupe, M.J., and Rudolph Micik.

World Health Organization. 1975. II. Special Subject. Children of School Age and Their Mortality and Hospital Morbidity Throughout the World. *World Health Statistics* **28**:140-53.

Young, W., and S. Smith, 1972. The Nature and Organization of Dental Practice. In Freeman, H., Levine, S., and L.G. Reeder, eds., *Handbook of Medical Sociology*. Englewood Cliffs, N.J.: Prentice-Hall.

Zahn, M. 1973. Incapacity, Impotence and Invisible Impairment: Their Effects Upon Interpersonal Relations. *Journal of Health and Social Behavior* **14**:115.

Glossary

Amalgam (dental) is an alloy of mercury with silver, copper, tin and zinc used to fill teeth.

Auxiliaries are ancillary personnel that assist the dentist by providing direct and indirect patient services as specified by dental laws and delegated by the dentist.

Calculus is calcified dental plaque which is hard and firmly attached to the teeth and other dental appliances that replace missing teeth.

Caries (dental) is a multifactorial disease of the teeth characterized by loss of minerals (decalcification) and accompanied or followed by disintegration of the organic matrix.

Debris is particulate unstructured matter loosely attached to the gums and teeth.

Deciduous dentition refers to primary, temporary, or baby teeth that are lost and replaced by permanent or adult teeth.

Dentate means having teeth or pointed conical tooth like projections.

DMF Score, a measure of dental caries experience, is the sum of decayed, missing and filled teeth (DMFT) or decayed, missing and filled tooth surfaces (DMFS).

Edentulous means without teeth.

Filled teeth are those diseased or traumatized teeth which have had decayed or missing parts replaced by appropriate dental materials to restore form and function.

Fluoridation is the adjustment of the fluoride content of a public central water supply to one part fluoride per one million parts of water, which is optimal for dental health.

Gerodontics (geriatric dentistry) is that branch of clinical dental practice dealing with the problems of aging, old age and senility peculiar to the oral cavity.

Gingivitis is an inflammation of the gingiva (gums).

Malocclusion refers to any deviation in the bite from the ideal contact of the maxillary (upper) teeth with the mandibular (lower) teeth.

Malposition is a deviation from the ideal tooth-to-tooth relationships occurring in either the maxillary (upper) or mandibular (lower) teeth.

Oral pathology is that branch of dentistry dealing with the structural and functional changes in oral tissues that cause or are caused by disease.

Orthodontic treatment (orthodontics) refers to the art and the science of the prevention and correction of dental and oral abnormalities and the malocclusion of teeth associated with dentofacial disharmonies.

Pedodontics is that branch of clinical dental practice dealing with the etiology, prevention, diagnosis and treatment of dental disorders of children.

Periodontal means of or pertaining to the state of health or disease of the periodontium, which is composed of the tissues that support the teeth.

Periodontal Index is a clinical measure of the extent and severity of those diseases which affect the supporting tissues of the teeth.

Periodontology is the art and science of the etiology, prevention, diagnosis and treatment of diseases of the supporting structures of the teeth.

Prophylaxis (dental) is the name for those dental procedures designed to remove soft and hard desposits that are irritants to the gums and to smooth and polish teeth surfaces to retard further formation of these local irritants.

Prosthesis (dental) is an appliance or device that replaces missing teeth and associated supporting oral structures.

Prosthodontics is the dental art and science of restoring function by replacing missing teeth and associated oral structures with artificial appliances.

Restorative care refers to the replacement of tooth structure lost through decay or accident using metallic, silicate or composite dental materials.

Restorative Index is the ratio of filled teeth to filled plus decayed teeth and is used to measure the dental care that has been provided in a community.

Simplified Oral Hygiene Index is a quantitative clinical measure of the cleanliness of the oral cavity that accounts for both soft and hard depsoits accumulated on teeth.

Stomatologist is a dentist with a broad biological background who treats disorders and diseases of the oral cavity and associated structures.

Index

About the Authors

Marcel A. Fredericks, professor of sociology, Loyola University of Chicago, received his Ph.D. in medical sociology from that institution. He established the Office of Research in Medical Sociology, at Loyola, and has since served as its director. Dr. Fredericks won a United States Public Health Service Fellowship for research and teaching at the Harvard University Medical School and was later appointed research associate in pediatrics there. With Dr. Mundy he is the author of *The Making of a Physician* and *The Sociology of Health Care*. In addition, he has published numerous professional articles.

Ralph R. Lobene, dean of the Forsyth School for Dental Hygienists in Boston and professor of dentistry and allied health there, earned his D.D.S. at the University of Buffalo as well as an M.S. degree from Tufts University. He has had experience in private dental practice, research and education and has published extensively in the fields of preventive dentistry and the delivery of dental care. He is the principal author of a recent Harvard University Press book, *The Forsyth Experiment; An Alternative System for Dental Care*, with the collaboration of Alix Kerr. He is a fellow of the International and American Colleges of Dentists.

Paul Mundy, professor of sociology, Loyola University of Chicago, received his Ph.D. with distinction from the Catholic University of America, where he later directed the undergraduate program in sociology. At Loyola he has been primarily responsible for developing its graduate program in sociology and has also served as department chairman. He has been editor of the *American Catholic Sociological Review* and president of both the American Catholic Sociological Society and the Religious Research Association. He is the coauthor of *The Making of a Physician* and *The Sociology of Health Care*.